AUDITORY   TECHNIQUES

Sponsored
by
The HEAR Foundation
in conjunction with
The San Diego Speech and Hearing Center
and Oralingua Staff

Proceedings of the
International Conference on
AUDITORY
TECHNIQUES

Edited by

CIWA GRIFFITHS, Ed.D.
Executive Director
The HEAR Foundation
Pasadena, California

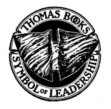

CHARLES C THOMAS • PUBLISHER
Springfield • Illinois • U.S.A.

Published and Distributed Throughout the World by
CHARLES C THOMAS • PUBLISHER
Bannerstone House
301–327 East Lawrence Avenue, Springfield, Illinois, U.S.A.

© *1974, by* CHARLES C THOMAS • PUBLISHER

ISBN 0–398–03047–2

Library of Congress Catalog Card Number: 73 18157

Printed in the United States of America

BB-14

PARTICIPANTS

Ole Bentzen, M.D.
State Hearing Center
Aarhus, Denmark

Ethel Cohen
Director
MICHA Center for Deaf Children
Tel Aviv, Israel

D.M.C. Dale, Ph.D.
Senior Lecturer in Education of the Deaf
London University
London, England

Rhea S. Das, Ph.D.
Professor
Department of Psychology
University of Wisconsin
Superior, Wisconsin

Allan Ebbin, M.D.
Genetics Division
Department of Pediatrics
USC Medical Center
Los Angeles, California

Judith Ebbin, M.A., M.S.
Assistant Research Director
HEAR Foundation
Pasadena, California

Leahea Grammatico, M.A.
Director
Peninsula Oral School for Death
Redwood City, California

Ciwa Griffiths, Ed.D.
Executive Director
HEAR Foundation
Pasadena, California

Tyler Hayes, M.A.
Speech and Hearing Specialist
Special Education Division
Los Angeles City School Districts
Los Angeles, California

Frances M. Kain
Teacher of Hearing-Impaired
Weisberg Memorial Center
Superior Public Schools
Superior, Wisconsin

Djordje Kostic, Ph.D.
Director
Institute for Experimental Phonetics and
*   Speech Pathology*
Belgrade, Yugoslavia

Agnes H. Ling, Ph.D.
Associate Director
McGill Project for Deaf Children
McGill University
Montreal, Canada

Enelda Luttmann
Director
Orientacion Infantil Para Rehabilitacion
*   Audiologica (O.I.R.A.)*
Mexico City, Mexico

Priscilla Pittenger Muir, Ed.D.
Department of Special Education
California State University
San Francisco, California

Kathryn O'Connor, B.A., M.Ed., M.A.
Supervisor
Program for the Hearing Impaired
Highline Public Schools
Seattle, Washington

Betty Petersen
Supervisor
Hearing Education Department
San Diego Speech and Hearing Center
San Diego, California

Doreen Pollack, B.A.
Director of Speech and Hearing
Porter Memorial Hospital
Denver, Colorado

Austin Riesen, Ph.D.
Department of Psychology
University of California
Riverside, California

Joseph Stewart, Ph.D.
Communication Disorders Specialist
Medical Services Branch
Dept. of Health, Education and Welfare
Alexandria, Virginia

Lois E. Tarkanian, M.A.
Director
Oralingua School for Deaf
Whittier, California

David Warren, Ph.D.
Department of Psychology
Riverside, California

Carroll White, Ph.D.
Naval Electronics Laboratory
San Diego, California

Robert Wieland, Ph.D.
Director
Exceptional Children's Center
Fort Lauderdale, Florida

CONTENTS

AUDITORY TECHNIQUES

GREETINGS

Dr. Griffiths: Welcome to the International Conference on Auditory Techniques. I already know that you are very intelligent people, that is why you came, so I know that these sessions are going to be well listened to, and hopefully each one of you will take home something that you can use to implement the whole idea of the auditory approach. So on behalf of the HEAR Foundation, its Board of Trustees and its Staff, we certainly welcome each and every one of you to this Conference.

The next person to speak to you is one of our cosponsors, Don Krebs of the San Diego Speech and Hearing Center. Dr. Krebs . . .

Dr. Krebs: Thank you, Dr. Griffiths. I want to welcome all of you here to our sunny southern California. Those of you who came early and met with all the rain that we had, we hadn't planned on that, but we planned four or five days of nice, clear, sunny weather. Those of you from the East who came out of the snow will notice that we keep ours up in the mountains where we can see it and not have to be concerned with it; however, if you like to ski, we do have some local ski areas that have a few feet of snow on them, I'm sure. It was with enthusiasm and anticipation that the San Diego Speech and Hearing Center accepted the cosponsorship of this program. I can't say that it has been an awful lot of work in cosponsoring it. We have given Dr. Griffiths a lot of verbal help, but I don't think we have done much of the physical labor that goes into conducting such a seminar.

For a number of years the San Diego Speech and Hearing Center has been rather active in sponsoring symposia specifically organized to explore philosophies, problems or techniques involving speech and hearing processes. These have been, indeed, significant challenges from which we have learned a great deal. More pointedly, however, we have, in some small measure, contributed to the knowledge of those attending the conferences.

This is the first International Seminar on Auditory Techniques, or on the Auditory Approach, and I hope it is just the beginning of many such seminars. Certainly, all of us assembled here today are keenly aware of the need for the contributions which will be forthcoming during the days which follow. Even cursory review of your program will reveal an excellent faculty assembled from the United States, Denmark, England, Yugoslavia, Canada and Mexico.

I feel that I speak for all of us, Dr. Griffiths, in wishing you the success

3

which this program deserves. Again, I speak for all of us who will be participating in this Conference in extending our thanks to all who made it a reality.

On behalf of the staff of the San Diego Speech and Hearing Center, welcome to this Conference on Auditory Techniques. May your tenure here be a rewarding one.

Dr. Griffiths: I now wish to introduce to you Lois Tarkanian, who is the Executive Director of the Oralingua School.

Lois Tarkanian: It is a pleasure and an honor for me this morning, as a representative of the teaching staff of Oralingua School, to share in welcoming you to this International Conference. Similarities are present in certain specifics of philosophies and methodologies, and all groups represented here today share a common bond of strong belief in the value of using the auditory pathways for hearing-impaired children. Each of us often has seen deaf children left unchallenged auditorily, their horizons limited. Too many of us currently are seeing lack of choices for parents who want their deaf children to achieve competent oral communication. It behooves each of us, who cares about the future of deaf children, to share our strength to insure that future children reach their highest possible functioning level. I want to say that all of us on the staff of Oralingua respect very much the efforts, the time and all the energy that Dr. Griffiths and workers at the HEAR Foundation have put into this Conference. I know it has been an magnanimous effort, and we are all excitedly looking forward to hearing all the speakers here today. We are very grateful that we have the opportunity to be able to attend.

Dr. Griffiths: Thank you, Mrs. Tarkanian. It gives me great personal pleasure to introduce the next speaker. I met Dr. Joseph Stewart, who is going to give our Keynote Speech, in Holland in 1961. Joe was so nice at that time because he walked to and from the meetings with me, and I didn't know when I went to Gronigen in 1961 that they had all cobble streets. I only took with me what was fashionable at that time which was three-inch heels. If you don't think that was noble of Joe to walk with me back and forth to those meetings! Of course I had to do it at a slow pace; therefore, he had to listen to what I had to say, and we became acquainted. Ten years later, who was it to whom I had to go to ask for support for an HEW contract but Joe Stewart. So you never can tell when you are going to meet people. And the nicest thing about Joe was that when I walked into his office ten years later he said, "Ciwa, you look exactly the same as ten years ago." Now that's the nicest thing you could ever say to a lady!

So not only was he my friend for that, but he has been the Director of our HEW contract which is winding up a three and one-half year period of study. You can tell by the program that he is a Communication Disorder Specialist of the Medical Services Branch of the Department of Health, Education and Welfare. Dr. Stewart . . .

Dr. Stewart: Thank you very much, Ciwa. I am glad to see that you remember those streets too; I still limp a little as a result of that experience. One of the advantages you have or prices you have to pay by being a civil servant is that you have the option, when you have the opportunity like this to get up and speak, of either submitting your remarks ahead of time for what they call clearance and having them appropriately laundered and looked over, or you have the option at the beginning of your speech of giving a disclaimer. So if you will all relax for a minute, I will rear back and lay a disclaimer on you, which is that nothing I say this morning necessarily reflects any policy of the Department of Health, Education and Welfare.

KEYNOTE SPEECH

WHEN ASKED IF I would be the keynote speaker for this Conference, I first asked myself the question, "What does a keynote speaker do?" In looking for the answer, I found that a keynote speaker can do a variety of things: He can, as we are all aware from recent events, extol the virtues of his political party and his candidate; or he can sing the praises of his own field of interests; less often, he will praise someone else's vested interest; often he reviews the literature so all the audience is on an equal footing; similarly, he can use his time to describe the *State of the Art;* unfortunately, he sometimes uses his opportunity to tell the audience what the speakers to follow are going to say; and, finally, he often is looked upon as a *cheerleader* to inspire his audience, the better to enable it to aspire to the lofty goals of the program to follow. Regardless of which technique is employed, however, you may rest assured that the keynoter is a strong adherent to the point of view of those who sought him for this purpose. The present keynoter is no exception. I do believe in the auditory approach being presented at this Conference, but I was not born with this point of view—it came slowly, at times somewhat grudgingly, but inexorably as the evidence of my senses overcame the rigidity of my preconceptions.

In preparing these remarks, then, it seemed that the uniqueness of this Conference, being international in scope and acknowledging that the problem of the hearing-impaired child extends beyond his ears, called for a combination of approaches in keynoting—with what I hope is not an undue emphasis on the *Cheerleader School of Oratory.*

When I left audiology as a practicing clinician eight years ago, one of my colleagues referred to me as an "angry young man." Now I find myself an "angry middle-aged man"—unfortunately still frustrated by the same things as before, including the snail's pace with which we seem to move toward solving the problems associated with hearing impairment in children.

For example, nearly twelve years ago, a conference similar to this one was held in The Netherlands. Of the 230 persons in attendance, only two had come from the United States. During the keynote address for that conference, the late Henk Huizing[1] had this to say:

> Impaired hearing in early childhood as a matter of fact involves a serious handicap, inasmuch as there exists a close relationship between the sense of hearing and the child's future intellectual level and its social consciousness.

[1] H.C. Huizing: Inaugural Address. *Proceedings of the Second International Course in Paedo-Audiology,* Groningen University, 1961.

Until shortly there existed no adequate means to liberate this handicapped child from its acoustic isolation.

Using this statement as our reference point, what progress can we account for in the twelve years since it was made? If twelve years seem too short a time, how then shall we measure our progress since the pioneers in the auditory approach began their work—Wedenberg, Whetnall, Pollack, Huizing, Bentzen and Griffiths established their programs in the late 1940's and early 1950's? To what extent can we say that their innovations are widely known, let alone widely used, especially in the United States?

The one major measure of progress that I do see is the more widespread use of hearing aids by the younger child. But while there may be more such aids in use, I do not see with this the accompanying methodology that the auditory approach requires. The major deficiencies that I see are these:

1. The aid itself is no *electronic penicillin,* no electronic wonder drug. Results of such studies as the recent one by Zink[2] on hearing aid stability should be kept constantly in mind if we are to insure maximal use of hearing aids by children. Zink's statement that "a significant number of hearing aids worn by children are functioning inefficiently" calls for us to demand a better product and a better procedure in *fitting* it.

2. The aid *by itself* cannot do the job. We do not expect a child to ride a bicycle the first time he gets on it, nor should we *expect* the child to become an *instant* hearing aid user, even though we often see this with infants.

3. Along with amplification, we need the methodology to provide the appropriate input, in appropriate amounts and throughout the spectrum of appropriate times. We also need to keep in mind the difference between the child's *hearing* age and his *chronological* age.

It seems to me that those of us in aural rehabilitation are faced with a number of paradoxes with which we must come to terms if we are to achieve the potential this field does—or should—have:

1. We rely both too much and too little on our instruments. We expect them to do nothing and we expect them to do everything.

2. We have what may be the world's greatest collection of unread scientific literature. It almost inevitably follows that we make little use of the knowledge from other areas—notably vision.

3. We know that audition is the first sense to develop, the only one which works full time and the last to go; yet, we immediately assume that if hearing is deficient, we must train the eyes to do the job. We know that the bulk of human learning is auditorily based and still we place children

[2] G.D. Zink: Hearing aids children wear. *Volta Rev,* 74:41–51, 1972.

in school on the basis of an *unaided* audiogram: We know that the child's hearing is much more acute, and his need for it much more acute than for the adult, yet we continue to apply hearing standards derived from the adult population to the infant and child.

A few weeks ago, for example, a document crossed my desk which blandly stated that a child's hearing loss must be *at least* 45 dB to be *significant*. What makes statements like this one particularly unfortunate, in my opinion, is that they tend to foster an orientation toward a looser, rather than stricter, definition of normality. We find in the Pittsburgh study,[3] for example, that the hearing acuity of children is such that the audiometers used were modified to test to −30 dB, the better to test that acuity. A 45 dB loss, to be *significant,* means we are willing to accept a true threshold loss of 74 dB— *significant,* indeed.

We are aware of the significance of a severe hearing loss, but what are some of the implications of our neglect of the *insignificant* hearing loss? In 1962, Eisen[4] reported that the child with early sensory deprivation, such as might result from otitis media, may never learn to listen, pay attention nor make auditory discriminations. As he matures, he does not have the foundation to develop implicit speech or thought—this in turn may lead to inadequate development of higher order abstraction and conceptualization. This may also have implications for reading difficulties. Superficially, the child may appear to be functioning normally. While there is not yet a substantial body of research literature to support these contentions fully, several studies do lend considerable support to this view: Holm and Kunze[5] for example, report that a group of children with chronic otitis media were found to be "significantly delayed in all language skills requiring the receiving of processing of auditory stimuli or the production of verbal responses." Ling and others[6] report that "Although . . . ear disease was not closely related to hearing for speech among Eskimo children, many surveys have shown that children with an extensive history of ear infections tend to be retarded in educational skills," a finding substantiated in an American Eskimo population. Kaplan and others,[7] in a study conducted in Alaska, report that "otitis media has been a significant cause of morbidity

[3] E.L. Eagles, S.M. Wishik, L.G. Doeffler, W. Melnick and H.S. Levine: Hearing sensitivity and related factors in children. Monograph, *Laryngoscope,* 1963.

[4] N.H. Eisen: Some effects of early sensory deprivation on later behavior: The quondam hard-of-hearing child. *J Ab Soc Psych,* 65:338–342, 1962.

[5] V.A. Holm and L.H. Kunze: Effect of chronic otitis media on language and speech development. *Pediatrics, 43:*833–839, 1969.

[6] D. Ling, R.H. McCoy, E.D. Levinson: The incidence of middle ear disease and its educational implications among Baffin Island Eskimo children. *Can J Pub Hlth,* 60:385–390, 1969.

[7] G.J. Kaplan, J.K. Fleshman, T.R. Bender, C. Baum and P.S. Clark: Long-term effects of otitis media: A ten-year cohort study of Alaska Eskimo children. Mimeographed report, 1970.

in Alaskan Eskimo children and its onset during the critical years of language development as well as the number of episodes play an important role in the impairment of verbal development."

These reports, plus others from neurophysiological literature, would seem to point up the old maxim from high school biology days—"use it or lose it." Certainly the work of Riesen, dating back to the 1940's, has terribly significant implications for us in the field of hearing—and yet, I must parenthetically ask, why is it only now that we are having an opportunity to hear of this work first-hand? To what might we attribute the cultural lag in replicating these visual studies to audition? On this point, several years ago an agency of the government held a small conference on auditory deprivation which was attended by a group of highly renowned neurophysiologists. One of the questions asked the group was: "What basis have we for assuming that auditory deprivation might produce effects similar to those demonstrated defects resulting from visual deprivation?" The answer given by the group was this: "What basis have you for assuming otherwise?"

This positive approach is matched by a statement included in the brochure announcing this Conference: "The auditory approach is a new science in the history of the deaf . . . but one which now has data, electronic equipment to use and techniques to report." I would hope that the Conference might have as one of its results the shifting of the burden of proof from those who maintain the auditory approach should be primary to those who maintain that it should not. For years I have heard the arguments raised that early amplification should not be tried for a variety of reasons—"it will only cause further hearing damage," "you shouldn't put a hearing aid on a child because he can't take care of it," "hearing aids are too expensive for children to use"—the arguments are endless.

On the point that hearing aids *may* cause further damage, I would like to quote from a former Surgeon General of the United States in remarks made during a conference in 1958 held on the problem of air pollution.[8] He said:

> Referring to the circumstantial evidence relating cancer to atmospheric pollution, I remarked that the case has not yet been proved. This legal metaphor is frequently used. I submit to you that it is misleading.
>
> In law, the suspect is innocent until his guilt has been proved beyond reasonable doubt. In the protection of human health, such absolute proof often comes late. To wait for it is to invite disaster, or at least to suffer unnecessarily through long periods of time.

[8] L. Burney: *Noise As a Public Health Hazard.* ASHA Reports #4, American Speech and Hearing Association, Washington, D.C., pp. 7–11, 1969.

I would say that proponents of the auditory approach need no longer feel that the burden of proof is on them.

The weight of all the available evidence is clearly on the side of this philosophy and the proponents of it should, as the Surgeon General noted in the case of air pollution, not wait for absolute proof. "To wait is to invite disaster . . . or to suffer unnecessarily through long periods of time."

To conclude, the sponsors of this Conference listed four dimensions by which to teach the hearing-impaired child to communicate—early intervention with carefully selected wide range amplification, full-time use of that amplification, constant exposure to normal speech and language and techniques to develop auditory processing. Quite obviously, we have the technology necessary to insure the wide use of instruments necessary to detect hearing loss early and provide the amplification necessary to help compensate for it. Equally as obvious, we have the techniques by which to provide the constant exposure to normal speech and language and develop auditory processing. The only step missing, it would seem, is the widespread acceptance of this approach and its implementation throughout the world. To this end, the present Conference makes a major contribution. This audience, by its very attendance, will play a major role in this development. I know you share with me concern that we not lose another generation of hearing-impaired children to our own ignorance, our own apathy and our devotion to the *status quo*. And now let us proceed to the business of the Conference.

JOSEPH STEWART, Ph.D.
Communication Disorders Specialist
Medical Services Branch
Department of Health, Education and Welfare

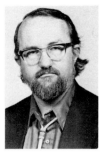

Dr. Stewart is Communications Disorders Specialist, Medical Services Branch, Indian Health Service. He was born in Salida, Colorado and received his B.A. from the University of Denver in 1949, his M.A. from that same university in 1950 and his Ph.D. from the University of Iowa, 1959. Dr. Stewart has held positions that include Research Associate, University of Iowa, 1958–59; Assistant Professor of Speech and Director of Hearing Center, University of Denver, 1959–65; Consultant Audiology and Speech Pathology, Neurological and Sensory Disease Control Program, U.S. Public Health Service, Rockville, Maryland, 1965–70.

Dr. Stewart is affiliated with the American Speech and Hearing Association; International Society of Audiology; Japan Audiological Society; Indian Speech and Hearing Association, International Society for General Semantics; Institute of General Semantics (Member, Board of Trustees); Founder, Wendell Johnson Memorial Library; All-India Institute of Speech and Hearing, Mysore, India; Library Chairman, Library Committee National Congress of American Indians. Dr. Stewart is listed in both *American Men of Science*, volume 11, 1967 and in *Who's Who in the South and Southwest*, Twelfth Edition, 1970.

Dr. Stewart's research work includes stuttering among North American Indians, effectiveness of educational audiology for young hearing-impaired children; inhibition facilitation of audition; audiometer design and calibration; otitis media in American Indian and Eskimo children; hearing aid need and utilization; presymptomatic speech characteristics in dysarthria; hearing loss and diabetes and pitch perturbation in laryngeal screening.

In addition to his time consuming work in research and administration, Dr. Stewart has to his credit a seemingly endless list of publications.

Chapter I

A CLINICAL GENETICIST VIEWS DEAFNESS*

ALLAN J. EBBIN
NANCY W. SHINNO

MANY PEOPLE in the United States are handicapped by hearing impairment which varies in severity from a mild loss to complete deafness. The causes of hearing loss are not completely known. About half of the deafness in children and about a third of the deafness in adults is considered genetic.

Prospective parents often consult the clinical geneticist about the risk of having an infant with a birth defect and the cause of the defect. They can be told that 2 to 4 percent of all newborns have a birth defect, that some of these defects are genetic and that others are acquired as the ·result of deleterious environmental influences. In most instances, a specific genetic or environmental cause cannot be identified. Acquired defects are not expected to recur in another pregnancy unless the same environmental influences are present. Many genetic defects may be expected to recur with a certain frequency depending on the mode of inheritance. Deafness present at birth (congenital deafness) can be either acquired or genetic. Most genetic forms of deafness are congenital, but some may appear later in life, for example, otosclerosis.

Acquired deafness may be the result of various factors occurring before, during or after birth. Before birth, maternal infections, such as rubella, may be transmitted to the fetus and cause deafness. At birth, factors such as prematurity, severe jaundice, trauma and infection may cause deafness. Later in life, meningitis, measles, mumps, noise and ototoxic drugs such as streptomycin, kanamycin and quinine may cause deafness.

The cause of deafness is often difficult to determine. If an individual has a congenital hearing loss alone and no family history of deafness, he could be deaf as the result of exposure to an environmental factor present *in utero* or soon after birth, or he could have a genetic form of deafness. A history of maternal infection, postnatal trauma or infection or a hearing loss occurring after the child has demonstrated the ability to hear is sug-

* Supported in part by Maternal and Child Health Service Grant Number 286.

gestive but not diagnostic of an acquired hearing loss. The relative frequency of the various causes of deafness is given in Table III-I.

The parents and other relatives of a deaf individual, the deaf person himself or a deaf couple may consult the clinical geneticist to determine the chance that deafness will recur in the family. Often people mistakenly believe that they have a high risk for having affected children when in reality they have no significant risk. If the chance of having a deaf child is high, such as one in two to one in four, many couples will decide not to have more children. They may prefer adoption. Some couples choose artificial insemination. If the risk is low, such as one in a hundred or less, some couples may take that risk. Some couples are more concerned about associated birth defects or mental retardation than deafness alone. They may feel that deafness is not a sufficiently severe handicap to limit their family size.

In order to establish the risks of recurrence, the geneticist requires a precise diagnosis, a family pedigree and accurate genetic information. He must be able to communicate effectively with the family to inform them of the risks of recurrence and the prognosis for the affected child.

A common misconception is that a person with no family history of deafness cannot have genetic deafness. This is not necessarily true. A negative family history is often found in recessive disorders. The child with a recessive form of deafness must inherit two mutant* genes for the same type of deafness, one from each parent. The carrier parent has only one gene for deafness and is normally hearing since two mutant genes must be present to cause the disorder. If two carrier parents mate, they have a 25 percent chance of having an affected child with each pregnancy. Everyone carries about five to ten mutant genes. If these mutant genes are rare, it is unlikely that carriers of the same mutant gene will mate and produce affected offspring. Consequently when parents are cousins or other blood relatives, the probability is increased that both of them will be carriers of the same mutant gene.

There are several different types of recessive deafness. If two parents are carriers of different types of recessive deafness, they have practically no chance of having a deaf child, since the child would not have a pair of the mutant genes. If the parents are affected with the same type of recessive deafness, all of their children are expected to be deaf.

If the deafness occurs as part of a genetic syndrome** with a known

---

* Mutant: a gene that has been altered from the normal state and may produce an abnormal condition.

** *Syndrome:* a group of symptoms or physical findings that occur together and characterize a disorder.

mode of inheritance, and if the syndrome can be readily identified, the risk of recurrence can be established. For example, Pendred's syndrome of congenital deafness and goiter is recessive and can be diagnosed by physical examination and thyroid function tests. The family can be informed that the child has a recessive condition and that each subsequent child would have a 25 percent risk of being affected.

Dominant forms of genetic deafness require only one mutant gene for their expression; therefore, a child with this type of deafness is likely to have a deaf parent from whom he inherited the mutant gene. Any offspring of an affected individual has a 50 percent chance of inheriting the mutant gene and would be deaf. Occasionally a child has a dominant form of deafness and two normal-hearing parents. In this instance we assume that a new gene mutation occurred in the child. Since the parents are not carriers of the mutant gene, they are at no increased risk of having another deaf child.

Genetic deafness may rarely have an X-linked recessive mode of inheritance. The mutant gene is on the X chromosome. A female would not be deaf unless her X chromosomes carried the mutant gene. This is unlikely. A male normally has only one X chromosome and a Y chromosome. If his X chromosome carries the mutant gene, it would not be counterbalanced by a normal X chromosome, and he would be deaf. He transmits this gene to none of his sons, who necessarily inherit his Y but not his X chromosome. He transmits the mutant gene to all of his daughters who inherit his X chromosome. These daughters are carriers. They have normal hearing since the mutant gene on one X chromosome is balanced by the other X chromosome. The male offspring of carrier women would have a 50 percent chance of inheriting the mutant gene in which case they would be deaf. The female offspring would have a 50 percent chance of inheriting the gene in which case they would be carriers.

When a deaf individual has deaf relatives, a family pedigree may indicate whether the deafness in the family is consistent with a recessive, dominant or X-linked mode of inheritance, and the counselor may inform the family of the risk of recurrence.

If the individual has other defects in addition to the deafness, it may be easier to make a precise diagnosis and determine the risk of recurrence. Such genetic syndromes include low set, malformed ears and conductive deafness, a recessive disorder; lack of skin pigment and nerve deafness in Waardenburg's syndrome, a dominant disorder; and craniofacial abnormalities and mixed nerve and conductive deafness in Treacher-Collins syndrome, also a dominant condition. Konigsmark (1969) divides sixty-two forms of genetic deafness into the following eight groups:

Group	Number
Hereditary deafness with no associated abnormalities	12
Hereditary deafness with external ear malformations	5
Hereditary deafness with skin disease	12
Hereditary deafness associated with eye disease	9
Hereditary deafness associated with nervous system disease	4
Hereditary deafness associated with skeletal disease	13
Hereditary deafness associated with kidney disease	3
Hereditary deafness associated with other abnormalities	4
Total	62

Chromosome disorders which occur in about one percent of all births are occasionally associated with hearing loss. For example, Trisomy D with an extra chromosome, Turner's syndrome with a missing chromosome and syndromes with a deletion of part of a chromosome may be associated with deafness. In these disorders the affected individuals have physical abnormalities and may have mental retardation. Many of these disorders are life threatening, and the affected child does not live long enough to manifest problems from deafness. Usually the parents show normal results from chromosome analysis and, therefore, have a very low risk of having another affected child. Rarely a parent may be a carrier of an abnormal chromosome and for this reason has an increased risk of having another affected child.

The audiogram can sometimes be of help in determining the type of deafness. The audiologist can distinguish between unilateral and bilateral involvement, between conductive and neural loss and between high and low frequency losses. In addition the use of serial audiograms will establish whether the loss is progressive. There are a few genetic disorders with typical audiometric patterns. For example, dominant progressive nerve deafness is a disease characterized by childhood onset of a progressive symmetrical neural loss beginning with high frequencies and leading to moderately severe high- and low-frequency loss in older age. Another example would be a dominant form of low-frequency hearing loss which is characterized by moderate neural low-frequency loss with slow pro-

gression to moderately severe neural loss involving all frequencies (Konigsmark, 1969).

Unfortunately, with present techniques, it is often impossible to determine the cause of deafness in an affected child with no associated birth
defects, no family history of deafness and no history of an environmental
cause. An exact diagnosis, a critical element in genetic counseling, is therefore not available, and a precise risk figure cannot be given.

In summary, when the cause of deafness is clearly understood, the
genetic counselor can inform the family of the risk of recurrence. Even
if he cannot give a precise risk figure, he may be able to allay parental
guilt about the cause of deafness and provide the family with a more
realistic basis for planning their child's treatment and determining their
family size.

REFERENCES

Fraser, G.R.: Profound childhood deafness. *J Med Genet, 1*:118–151, 1964.
Konigsmark, B.W.: Hereditary deafness in man. *NEJM, 281*:713–720, 774–778, 827–
832, 1969.

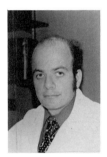

ALLAN J. EBBIN, M.D.

Allan Ebbin is presently associated with Los Angeles County-University of Southern
California Medical Center, where he is Assistant Professor of Pediatrics and Assistant
Director of the Genetics Division. He received his undergraduate training at New
York University and his medical education at the State University of New York-
Upstate Medical Center. His internship and residency in pediatrics were at the Los
Angeles County-University of Southern California Medical Center. When associated
with the Center for Disease Control, Atlanta, Georgia, he established the first birth
defects registry in the United States. His major professional interests are in the area
of birth defects, epidemiology and genetic counseling. Dr. Ebbin, a frequent con-
tributor to professional journals and participant in numerous conferences, is a Fellow
of the American College of Pediatrics. He serves as consultant to the Los Angeles
County Health Department and the National Foundation for birth defects.

Chapter II

EARLY IDENTIFICATION—PLUS
THE AUDITORY APPROACH

CIWA GRIFFITHS

ALMOST FORTY years ago, I met the first deaf child to enter my life. Little did I know that she would key my future so that, years later, I would stand before a group such as this to report some vital experiences which led to significant information and the implementation of that information.

At the time that I entered the field of the education of the deaf, hearing aids were *not* taken for granted; in fact, few individual aids were used by deaf children. The group hearing aids in schools for the deaf were used for part of the school day, but the deaf child lived in a world of silence most of the time. Yet, when I visited schools for the deaf, I was told that the child who had the better and more intelligible speech had more hearing than the others. Even then, my thought was that a change in hearing could be effected by the use of an aid which would give the profoundly deaf child more sound with which to work.

Years would go by while I worked with many deaf children, always using an aid and always seeking a way to keep the child in the mainstream with his hearing peers. And some children were able to do that years ago when hearing aids were not the same and when the idea was not always accepted readily by the parents or by the school.

When, over twenty years ago, I had insight regarding early intervention during the first three years of life which would take advantage of a maturation period of listening and learning to talk, I was really in hot water! At that time, I was not aware that anyone else had already started with a similar viewpoint.

To the late Dr. Edith Whetnall, I owe a great deal of inspiration. In 1954 when I studied with her in London at the Audiology Unit of the National Throat, Nose and Ear Hospital, it was my first professional experience in discussions which created compatible excitement.

To my friends, Margaret and Glen Bollinger, I, and many deaf children everywhere, owe an incalculable debt for their support, both financial and moral, which made the HEAR Foundation possible. And even to those who have been critical of the HEAR Foundation, I owe something: once I become angry, obstinate and determined, nothing can stop me!

As the years of children, work and inquiry have succeeded one another, I found out what I did not know . . . and it was a great deal. But problems present a reason for inquiry, and inquiry leads to answers.

The following factors are, in my opinion, of prime importance in the auditory approach.

Early Identification

Early identification of hearing problems is certainly possible and relatively easy, if one has the opportunity of seeing the infants. There are many critical indices which give important information from which diagnosis of hearing levels can be made. As important as the *routine* screening of hearing of newborns is that that procedure is still in the future. That it should be done is logical and critical. This area of science is waiting for the development of an adequate, objective tool to measure response to sound. With the realization of such instrumentation, I believe such routine testing would be quickly adopted. The medical profession has for some time been working in areas of early development; prenatal studies and early deprivation studies are no longer rare.

Instrumentation

The Evoked Response Audiometers have been used for a number of years in many centers; much information has been gathered through this means of testing. Studies of heart rate response are now being pursued in a number of centers, of which we are one. At the HEAR Foundation, we have gathered important data in the administration of the cardiac response test. We have demonstrated the fact that the heart rate will usually decelerate with threshold sound within four to six seconds after onset of signal and will accelerate to high intensity signals. The Cardiac Digital Audiometer with its print-out information is our newest tool. It needs to be validated in a hospital setting. We now have a prototype of a Digital Cardiac Audiometer which is currently being used at a medical center.

What I am endeavoring to do at this time is to produce a piece of equipment which will accurately and instantly report the state of the infant in response to sound stimuli, be a piece of equipment that a technician can use in a hospital environment where there is no sound room . . . and, oh yes, be something that is not too expensive.

Early Intervention

Our years of work have consistently demonstrated the advantage of early intervention. (Mrs. Ebbin will later in this program report on the critical age of hearing.) The youngest baby was 21 days of age when fitted with hearing aids. We have had a total of about 150 infants of less than one year.

Binaural Fitting

Since 1956, the HEAR Foundation has routinely fitted the children with binaural aids. We know that (1) the children accept their aids for full time wearing almost immediately; (2) they have the ability to localize sound and therefore separate speech from background noise increasing the clarity of sounds; (3) they better orient themselves in their environment in space relationships; (4) both neural pathways are utilized; and (5) different hearing acuity levels can be adequately fitted.

Full Time Wearing of Aids

Hearing aids should be worn full time. Only for safety factors for the young child should aids be removed for sleeping or for allowing the ear canals to *breathe*. Sometimes this latter need is satisfactorily cared for by sleeping with an aid in one ear one night and the other the next. Many of the HEAR Foundation children, from two or three years on, insist in sleeping with their aids.

Wearing hearing aids all day begins from the time the aids are first put on. It is essential that the child be supplied with amplified sound for the maximum number of hours.

Wide Range Amplification

As hearing aids pass only those sounds between 300 to 3000 cycles (or some from 100 to 3000 cycles) in a limited frequency range, the deaf child has a nasal tone to his voice and has difficulty in the discrimination and production of many consonant sounds.

The HEAR Foundation developed the HEAR Training Unit (HTU I) and then the HTU II for the purpose of having a clinical instrument which will provide wide range (40 to 17,000 cycles) and therefore provide amplification which more nearly resembles normal hearing. This amplifying system has the further advantage of supplying on a prescription basis a compensatory amplifying system for each child. In addition, formant cards allow the child to hear each sound in isolation and to be able to reproduce that sound through audition.

The HEAR Foundation has also developed the HEAR III, an individual unit with the same frequency characteristics, i.e. range from 40–17,000 cycles. It has the advantage of being set for the individual's loss and is small enough to be carried to school and therefore worn in the classroom as well as at home. The number of extra hours to which the child is exposed to wide range amplification is thereby greatly increased.

The next goal is to finish the development of a small, wearable aid with wide range, prescriptive characteristics. Full time wearing of such amplifying devices would make a significant difference in acquiring speech and language.

Teaching Techniques

The auditory approach appropriately calls for new teaching techniques. Establishment of rate and rhythm of speech, inflection and auditory skills of discrimination are basics. No longer is articulation the greatest concern but rather language learned in a natural way and articulation refined through the ability to hear and repeat sounds. Concentration on using every remnant of residual hearing is paramount to develop adequate auditory processing.

Hearing Environment

An environment of normal speech and language is essential to the eventual acquisition of normal speech and language. Where it is possible for the child to pursue his academic education with those who hear normally, he should be full time in a normally-speaking world. If the child is taught to repeat through hearing, the eventual result is to repeat what his environment provides.

Classroom Teacher Orientation

The deaf child who used to be isolated in a deaf world need no longer exist. But the child with aids who is a member of a regular classroom is not the only one who needs expert assistance. The classroom teacher needs orientation to the special child. Routine evaluation of progress of the child should be made possible with evaluative techniques pertinent to the problem. The classroom teacher should be given the assistance needed and should be alerted to the child's abilities not his limitations, if any.

Learning Disabilities

The increasing knowledge of the existence of learning disabilities of the normally hearing has its value in relating to the reality of learning disabilities being present with hearing problems. Many techniques have been developed to improve the teaching for learning disabilities; they are also appropriate for the deaf child with learning disabilities. More critical is the need to identify such problems at the onset in order that dual programs can be of assistance to the child before permanent problems are irreversible.

Summary

In summary, much that has been learned over the years in the HEAR Foundation program has immediate application and should be used to realize the fullest potential of the hearing-handicapped child. But there is still more to be done. At least three areas should be explored and developed to add to the efficiency and results of the auditory approach: (1) early identification of other problems which influence the child's learning abilities and appropriate techniques to be employed; (2) the development of wide range, prescriptive, wearable hearing aids; and (3) a team-work approach between those persons interested in the welfare of children: parents, therapists, special schools and regular schools at every level. The presence of this number of personnel attending the International Conference on Auditory Techniques indicates interest. From *interest* should come the solution.

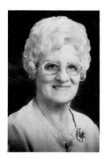

CIWA GRIFFITHS, Ed.D.

A.B. San Francisco State College, 1932
Teacher, one room school, Monterey County, California, 1937–40
Graduate study, Special Education, Summer Session, 1939, University of California, Berkeley, California
Teacher-in-training, Clarke School for the Deaf, Northampton, Mass., 1940–41
M.S. in Education, Science, Massachusetts University, 1941
Teacher of the Physically Handicapped and Elementary Supervisor, Monterey County Schools, California 1941–44
Graduate Student in Administration, University of California at Berkeley, California, 1942
Consultant in Education of Hard-of-Hearing, State of California Department of Education, 1944
Lecturer in Special Education, Summer Session, Stanford University and San Francisco State College, 1944
Coordinator of Special Education, San Diego County Schools, San Diego, California, 1944–51
Lecturer, Special Education, Summer Sessions: San Diego State College, 1945 and 1949; Vassar College, 1947 and 1948

Consultant, P.S. 47, Experimental Pre-School Program, New York City, 1948–54

Tutor, John Tracy Clinic, 1950–51

Assistant Professor of Education, Special Education, Los Angeles State College, 1951–54

Study, Audiology Unit, Royal National Throat, Nose, and Ear Hospital, London, England, 1954

Ed. D., University of Southern California, Los Angeles, California 1955

Executive Director, HEAR Foundation, Pasadena, California 1954–

Lecturer, Ocidental College, Los Angeles, California 1958–

Project Director, HEW Study Contract, 1969–72

> Project Officer, Joseph L. Stewart, Ph.D., Neurological and Sensory Disease Control Program, Division of Chronic Disease Programs

MEMBER: Delta Epsilon, University of Southern California
>   American Speech and Hearing Association
>   Council for Exceptional Children
>   Quota Club International

HONORARY MEMBER:
>   Zeta Phi Eta

>   INTERNATIONAL CONFERENCE PARTICIPATION BY INVITATION
>   1. II International Audiology Conference
>   Panel: Neonatal Testing
>   Copenhagen, Denmark, 1964
>   2. The Young Deaf Child: Identification and Management
>   Toronto, Canada 1964
>   3. International Conference on Oral Education of the Deaf
>   Northampton, Massachusetts, 1967
>   4. International Congress on the Education of the Deaf
>   Stockholm, Sweden, 1970

>   NATIONAL CONFERENCE PARTICIPATION BY INVITATION
>   1. Alexander Graham Bell Association National Meeting, Salt Lake City, 1964
>   2. ASHA: A Conference on Hearing Aid Evaluation Procedures, Chicago, 1967
>   3. Short Course: ASHA Annual Convention, Chicago, 1969
>   4. Conference on Newborn Hearing Screening: California State Department of Health, Bureau of Maternal and Child Health, San Francisco, 1971

PUBLICATIONS:

"Patterns," 1944, Crown Publications

"The Utilization of Individual Hearing Aids on Young Deaf Children," a dissertation presented to the faculty of the School of Education, the University of Southern California, June 1955

"Conquering Childhood Deafness," 1967, Exposition Press

"Til forever is Past," 1967, Exposition Press

CALIFORNIA CREDENTIALS:
1. General Junior High
2. General Elementary
3. Special Credential to Teach the Hard-of-Hearing
4. Special Secondary Credential to Teach the Deaf
5. Special Secondary Credential to Correct Speech Defects
6. Supervision in Elementary Education
7. Supervision in the Field of Hearing

Chapter III

VISUAL TESTING WITH EVOKED POTENTIALS*

Carroll T. White

INTRODUCTION

THE DEVELOPMENT of average response computers has made it possible to detect the minute changes in the electrical activity of the brain brought about by the presentation of sensory stimuli. The electrical activity is obtained by placing electrodes at appropriate locations on the scalp. The complex ongoing activity thus obtained (the electroencephalogram or EEG) contains a great deal more than the desired responses to the stimuli. The extraneous activity is effectively averaged out by summing the responses to a number of stimulus presentations. It is assumed that what remains after this procedure is in some way related to the stimulus which has been presented and/or to the subject's perceptual reaction to that stimulus.

The described approach forms the basis of obtaining auditory-evoked potentials (AEP) which are widely used for obtaining hearing thresholds. In a similar manner responses of the tactile sense (somatosensory-evoked potential, or SEP) and the visual sense (visual-evoked potential, or VEP) can be obtained. A detailed treatment of the theory, techniques and findings in this area of research is contained in the recent book by Regan (1972). The present paper presents a brief review of the basic studies which laid the groundwork for visual testing using this approach and refers to reports not covered by Regan, which detail the ways in which the VEP is being used clinically.

In all of the examples presented in this paper, a single electrode was placed on the midline of the scalp about one inch forward of the inion, directly over the visual cortex. In most cases a relatively large number of

* The review of basic studies contained in this paper was first presented at the NASA Conference on evoked potentials held in San Francisco, California, on September 10–12, 1968. The proceedings of that conference were published under the following title: Donchin, E. and Lindsley, D.B. (Eds.): *Average Evoked Potentials: Methods, Results and Evaluations.* NASA AP–191, Washington, D.C., U.S. Government Printing Office, 1969.

23

individual responses were summed to obtain the waveforms shown, usually 50 or 100, but such a large number would not be needed in actual usage. The papers in the Bibliography must be referred to for more detailed descriptions of the techniques involved in the actual application of this method of testing.

Review of Basic Studies

Figure III-1 presents VEPs from two individuals responding to four different types of patterns. At the top is a checkerboard; the second stimulus is a horizontal grating in which the distance between the black lines is about the same as the width of the *checks* in the checkerboard. The third stimulus is a group of concentric circles, and the last is a set of radial lines.

PATTERN

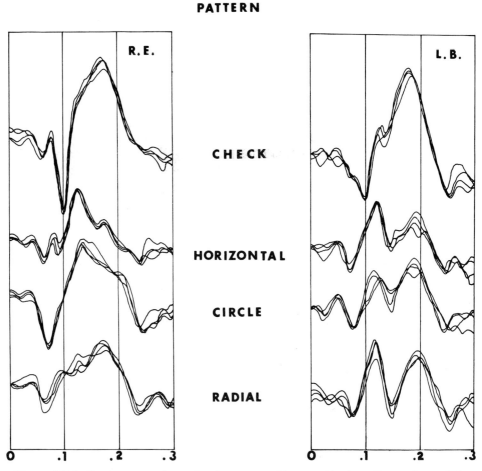

Figure III-1. Responses to four visual patterns. Four replications for each condition, N = 100 for each replication. Binocular stimulation (negative down).

There were four replications on successive days, and 100 stimuli in each replication. There is a high degree of intrasubject reliability; note also that there is much intersubject variability, its degree depending upon the type of pattern.

The radial lines elecited quite a different pattern in the two subjects. It turned out that there was a good reason for this; one subject was badly astigmatic, and the other was not.

We subsequently conducted a study of the effect of the size of the checks in a checkerboard on the VEP. A similar study was conducted by Rietveld and his associates (Rietveld *et al.*, 1967). Figure III-2 presents some of the results of this study. The bottom record was elicited by a pattern with

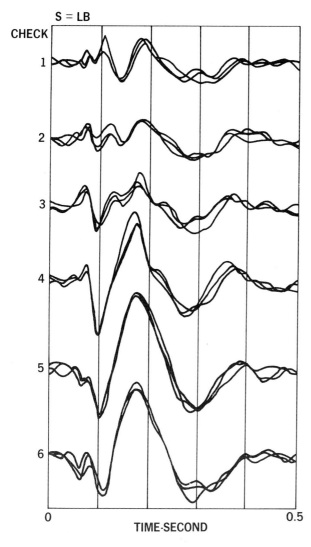

Figure III-2. Evoked potential and check size. Largest checks at top of record. In *Check* 5 each unit subtended 10 min of arc; N = 50 per record. Binocular stimulation (negative down).

5 minutes of arc per unit check, the next about 10, then 20, 40 and so forth. The independent variable is thus the density of the contour. As contour density increases, there is a very striking increase in the amplitude of response. Note that the increase in amplitude is most marked at the 100-msec point and at about 180 msec.

These data corroborate the findings of Rietveld and his associates very well. We also find, as they do, that there is a size of the checkerboard element that elicits a maximum VEP, and that it subtends a visual angle of about 10 minutes of arc.

Figure III-3 introduces another aspect of the work. This, and Figure III-4, represent work previously reported by Harter and White (1968). Subjects were presented with a checkerboard of the optimum design, elements of 10 to 15 minutes of arc. The stimuli were presented in focus and

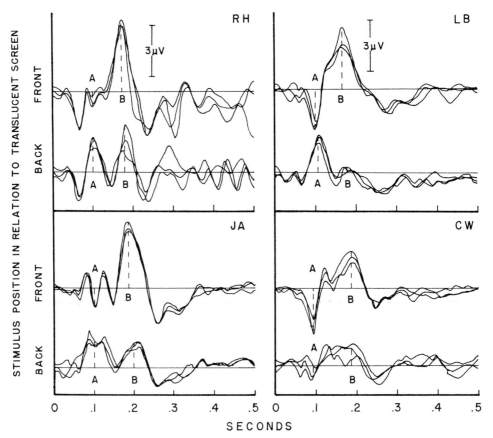

Figure III-3. Responses to sharply focused (front) and blurred (back) images for four subjects; N = 100 per record. Binocular stimulation (negative down).

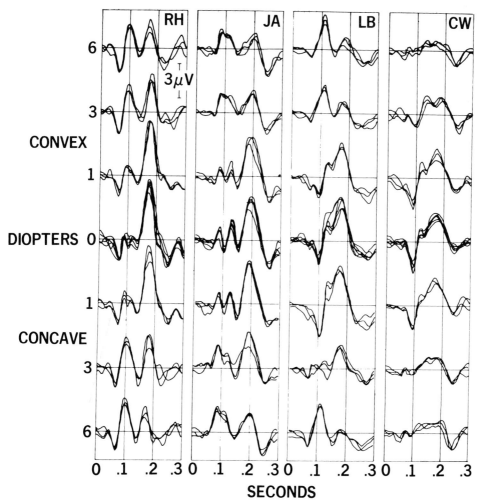

Figure III-4. Change in responses of four subjects as a function of degree of sharpness of contour in a visual pattern. Most clear around 0 diopters, badly blurred at both extremes (+ 6 and − 6 diopters). N = 100. Presentation rate 1/second. Binocular stimulation. Negative down.

out of focus to four subjects. The records labeled *front* were obtained when a transparency was placed in front of the diffusing milk-glass light window, while *back* indicates that we placed it behind the milk glass. The front condition produced a clear, sharply-defined image, while the back condition caused a badly blurred image of the checkerboard.

Again there were individual differences, but there were components common to all subjects (we have labeled them A and B). Rietveld and his associates discovered essentially the same two components and called them Gamma and Z. The A is a negative intrusion that occurs at about 100 msec after the flash when there is contour present, and it seems that the amplitude of the negative intrusion is related to both the amount and quality of contour (the sharpness of the contour). Our A, in this figure, appears for every individual. Its amplitude peaks when the stimulus is in focus. In subject LB, an actual inversion can be seen from negativity to positivity, depending on whether the stimulus is in focus or out of focus. In the case of CW, the curve never goes positive. (This has since been learned to be due to marked individual differences shown in response to patterns presented to the upper and the lower visual fields.)

Component B is most positive at 180 msec when the stimulus is in focus. This was true in four subjects and in all the replications. We have replicated this study with about 40 to 50 subjects in the past year, and we have generally obtained the same results.

Figure III-4 shows results obtained when ophthalmic lenses were used to defocus the image in gradual steps, from 1 to 6 diopters. You can see the gradual shift in both the A and B components.

There is evidence that these components are definitely neurogenic and that they are visually specific. These components can only be recorded from a very restricted area of the scalp over the occipital cortex. If you record at the inion, on the midline and towards the vertex in small steps, a certain point is reached about 2 inches forward of the inion where these components will disappear. It is a marked and sharp break.

We assume that when we present a very complex figure, such as the checkerboard, that the VEP we record is the sum of the responses to flashes of light per se, perhaps some non-specific response, and thirdly the response to the contour that was presented. We were only interested in the contour response. We thought it feasible to eliminate all of the other components by obtaining a set of responses and then subtracting the responses to unpatterned light. We thus completely defocussed the image and subtracted, by means of the computer, the same number of flashes that we used with the various checkerboard stimuli. Under these circumstances, we hoped to obtain a better estimate of the contribution of the contour only.

Figure III-5 shows an example of the subtracting process. At the top left is the standard response of a normal adult to a sharply focused checkerboard of optimum size; below it are the responses obtained using lenses of 1, 3 and 6 diopters. On the right side of the figure are records from which we have subtracted responses to 50 flashes, with —10 diopter lenses before each eye. At 6 diopters, the record appears to be about at the noise level of the system.

Figure III-6 shows the effects of astigmatism on the VEP of a subject. A grating of fine black lines was presented at different angles—first hori-

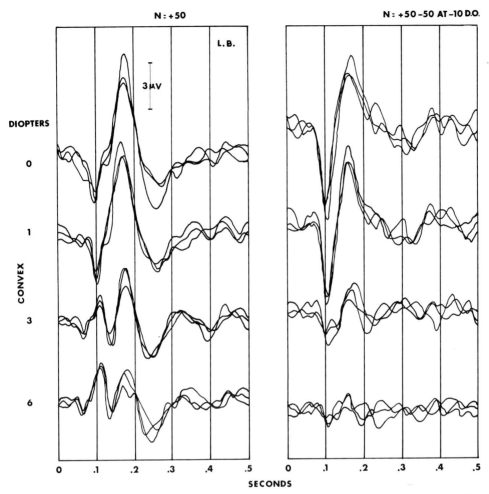

Figure III-5. Example of subtraction technique. Original records are at left. At right are the results after an equal number of responses to a stimulus with no contour information have been subtracted. Binocular stimulation. Negative down.

zontal, then up to the right, then vertical and then up to the left. If you know what to look for, you can immediately see that one of these is better than the others; however, the subtraction technique makes it very clear. Good responses were obtained when the grating was horizontal; we obtained just noise otherwise. Under these circumstances, this person could only see the lines when they were horizontal, or 5° or 6° off horizontal. Anything else appeared completely blurred to him.

He is an ideal subject because his right eye does not have any appreciable astigmatism. The right side of the figure shows the response to right-eye stimulation at horizontal, 45°, 90° and 135°. After subtraction, the

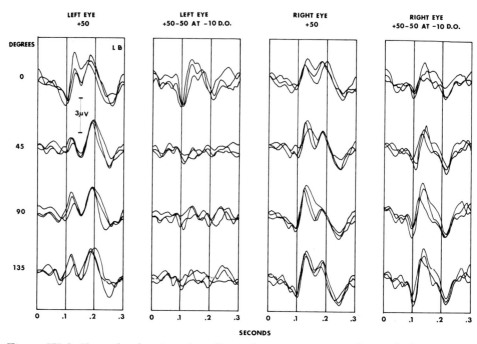

Figure III-6. Example showing the effect of ·astigmatism on the evoked response. Stimulus was a grating pattern consisting of fine black lines. Subject had marked astigmatism in the left eye and a very slight amount in the right eye. Negative down.

largest response was at 135°; next highest was at 90°, next at 45° and the lowest at the horizontal. His perceptual response verified this. He could see all of these lines very clearly, but the highest contrast was at 135° and gradually decreased to a medium gray. The optometrist who studied him for us agreed with this but said that the degree of astigmatism present in his right eye was so slight that he would not bother to correct it.

Clinical Applications

The results of the studies just described, and of others like them, made it clear that the VEP was potentially valuable as a clinical testing procedure. As a result of these results being made known to optometric and ophthalmological groups, in-depth evaluations were carried out to establish clinical procedures to be followed and to establish normative data.

One major evaluative study was carried out by the U.S. Army (Duffy and Rengstorff, 1971). In this study the results of the earlier work were verified and extended. Detailed plans were also presented for completely automating the visual testing process. The other major evaluation of the VEP technique was carried out at the Optometric Center of New York

(Ludlam and Meyers, 1972). This work was specifically oriented toward developing procedures for the testing of young children. This group now routinely carry out refractions on 12-month-old patients.

Other work being done at various laboratories indicates that the technique might be useful with much younger children. It is hoped that the technique can be modified for children just a few months old so that visual screening procedures can be instituted, allowing visual problems to be detected before permanent impairment of vision occurs. The technique has already been shown to be able to detect amblyopia in young children (Lombroso *et al.*, 1969). This could prove eventually to be the most valuable application of the VEP. The more subtle effects of the relative sensory deprivation produced by blurred vision during critical periods of the brain's maturing process must also be considered.

Table III-I*

Causes of Deafness		Percentage
Genetic:	(Recessive	37.5
	(Dominant	12.5
	(Sex-linked	1.5
Acquired:	(Prenatally	6.0
	(Perinatally	10.0
	(Postnatally	30.0
Congenital malformations (includes chromosomal and other disorders not listed above)		2.5

*Adapted from Fraser, G.R.: Profound childhood diseases. *J Med Genet*, 1:118–151, 1964.

SELECTED BIBLIOGRAPHY

Duffy, F.H. and Rengstorff, R.H.: Ametropia measurements from the visual evoked response. *Amer J Optom and Arch Amer Acad Optom*, 48: 717–728, 1971.

Harter, M.R. and White, C.T.: Effects of contour sharpness and check-size on visually evoked cortical potentials. *Vision Res*, 8:701–711, 1968.

Lombroso, C.T., Duffy, F.H. and Robb, R.M.: Selective suppression of cerebral-evoked potentials to patterned light in amblyopia. *Electroenceph Clin Neurophysiol*, 27:238–247, 1969.

Ludlam, W.M. and Meyers, R.R.: The use of visual-evoked responses in objective refraction. *Trans NY Acad Sci*, 34:155–170, 1972.

Millodot, M. and Riggs, L.A.: Refraction determined electro-physiologically. *Arch Ophthalm*, 84:272–278, 1970.

Regan, D.: *Evoked Potentials in Psychology, Sensory Physiology and Clinical Medicine.* New York, John Wiley and Sons, 1972.

Rietveld, W.J., Tordoir, W.E.M., Hagenouw, J.R.B., Lubbers, J.A. and Spoor, Th.

A.C.: Visual evoked responses to blank and to checkerboard flashes. *Acta Physiol Pharmacol Neerl, 14:*259–285, 1967.

White, C.T.: Evoked cortical responses and patterned stimuli. *Amer Psychol, 24:*211–214, 1969.

White, C.T.: The visual evoked response and patterned stimuli. In Newton, G. and Riesen, (Eds.): *Advances in Psychobiology,* Vol. II. New York, John Wiley and Sons, (In Press).

White, C.T. and Bonelli, L.: Binocular summation in the evoked potential as a function of image quality. *Amer J Optom Arch Amer Acad Optom, 47:*304–309, 1970.

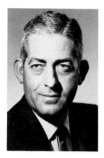

CARROLL T. WHITE, Ph.D.

Dr. Carroll T. White is an experimental psychologist in the Human Factors Division at Naval Electronics Laboratory Center, San Diego.

He holds a BSEE degree from Rice Institute, Houston, Texas; a B.A. in Psychology from University of Arizona; an M.S. Degree in Psychology from Brown University, Providence, R.I. and a Ph.D. in Experimental Psychology, also from Brown University. He received his doctorate after completing one year on campus at Providence under NELC's Advanced Study Plan.

Dr. White has authored over 40 professional papers, primarily in the fields of vision and visual perception. Most of these papers have appeared in the *Journal of the Optical Society,* the *Journal of Experimental Psychology* and *Science.*

He is a member of Sigma Xi, a science honorary, and Phi Kappa Phi, a university honorary. Additionally, he holds membership in the Human Factors Society of America and is listed in *American Men of Science* and the *International Dictionary of Biography.*

Dr. White holds a patent for "Cross-Polarized Lighting Techniques for Improving Operations of Cathode-Ray Tube Displays" and has a joint patent pending with Dr. M. Russell Harter on "Cortical Response Method of Computing Degree of Visual Aberration." He received the NELC award for Scientific Achievement (1968) the San Diego Creativity Society Award (1969) and Gentlemen of Distinction (Temple Beth) (1970).

Chapter IV

STUDIES OF EARLY SENSORY DEPRIVATION IN ANIMALS

Austin H. Riesen

Most experimental studies of early sensory deprivation have for obvious reasons been done with vision and on animals. The eyes are more easily occluded than are any other sense organs, and removal of the restriction for later behavioral testing or for permitting use of the sense mode prior to physiological and anatomical evaluations is easily accomplished. There has been just enough study of auditory and other kinds of sensory deprivation to permit us to say that the rather dramatic evidence for an early sensitive period may not be characteristic solely of the visual sensory system.

The loss of a sense organ results in transneuronal degenerative changes. Brain regions so deprived of input have for some time been known to undergo cellular losses (Riesen, 1966). Changes that result from disuse proceed more slowly, perhaps, and only in the past 20 years have such changes been established beyond reasonable doubt. Neurochemical studies have shown that disuse actually results in changes in nerve cell metabolism within a fraction of an hour. Initially, these are readily reversed, however, and therefore only longer term studies can provide the necessary data to determine whether critical or sensitive periods of growth and functional development are involved.

Visual Deprivation

During the decade of the sixties, the studies of kittens undergoing monocular visual deprivation dramatized an early critical period for the development and stabilization of pattern vision (Dews and Wiesel, 1970). Occlusion of one eye during the period from four weeks to twelve weeks of age results in a permanent loss of visual acuity and a behavioral blindness that is only very slowly and only partially recoverable during subsequent years even when the occlusion is shifted to the other eye in order to force the use of the earlier deprived eye. Very little and only temporary effects are produced if the same procedure is followed after normal use of both eyes to the age of twelve weeks. Similar results, but with indications of a somewhat longer sensitive period, have been found in young rhesus monkeys (von Noorden, Dowling and Ferguson, 1970). A much less drastic deprivation procedure is to allow each eye to see patterns part of each day when the other is occluded. This preserves form vision within a given eye, but the result when monocular exposures are continued through the sensitive developmental period is an animal that loses its stereoscopic depth perception and may show an alternating strabismus.

More extensive deprivation that is imposed by exclusion of all light produces a marked retardation of development of the visual system followed by cellular atrophy at some levels. In primates the ganglion cell layer of the retina eventually loses most of its nerve cells and shrinks to a small fraction of its normal thickness. Other layers may also become thinner and show reductions in the total RNA (ribonucleic acid) contents of the cells, without loss of cell numbers (Rasch, Swift, Riesen and Chow, 1961). Whether recovery can occur, and to what extent, depends on several factors: species of animal, duration of deprivation and age at onset of deprivation.

In spite of total darkrearing, certain visually guided behaviors may appear immediately when the deprivation period is ended, thus providing sound evidence that such behaviors are innately organized. No prior experience, for example, is necessary for laboratory rats to show visual depth avoidance after darkrearing to 60 or 90 days. Still longer darkrearing temporarily abolishes this behavior, and a period of 20 days or more in normal light may be required to restore it. Darkrearing delays the onset of the b-wave of the ERG (electroretinogram) and retards the normal development of the cortical evoked response.

If a milder form of deprivation, rearing under diffused light is imposed binocularly, the elaboration during early development of late components of the visual-evoked response to patterns, such as Doctor White has just described, is prevented. Cats and chimpanzees so deprived learn luminous flux discriminations readily, but these animals require many more trials to learn complex form discriminations or the discrimination of stimulus movement from nonmovement. The effects of pattern deprivation are thus, not surprisingly, confined to behaviors that depend upon pattern recognition. These include orientation of the animal and the coordination of the two eyes, visual pursuit of moving patterns and the discrimination of moving from nonmoving patterns. All of these uses of vision are impaired by early pattern deprivation. Subsequent development of appropriate behavior proceeds much more slowly after the deprivation has been maintained during the sensitive period. Results for different animals are also more variable. Some cats require four or five times longer than others to develop normal discriminations or coordinations, and a few fail to reach the equivalent of normal performances in over a year's time in fully visible surroundings. Carefully paced encouragement or *forced* use of visual guidance seems to be needed, and this may have to be tailored to the individual animal. Aggressive cats learn much for themselves, while timid ones make no progress without some intervention. (Cf. Baxter, 1966; Riesen, 1958.)

Auditory Deprivation

By keeping one group of rats in a sound shielded room at sound levels below 15 decibels for eight months from birth and comparing these with animals living in noise that fluctuated between 40 and 80 decibels, a group of experimenters produced evidence for reduced sensitivity to sound following partial auditory deprivation (Batkin, Groth, Watson and Ansberry, 1970). Evoked potentials were used to demonstrate the raised threshold. Some recovery by *some* of the deprived animals was found to occur after three weeks in a greater sound field.

By increasing or decreasing auditory stimulation in duck embryos, Gottlieb (1971) was able to accelerate or delay the normal time after hatching at which the ducklings first recognized the maternal call of their own species as distinct from that of other species.

Quite analogous to the effects of visual pattern deprivation are some data on auditory deprivation reported by Tees (1967). He reared rats in sound attenuation chambers and with ear plugs. Following a deprivation period from shortly after birth to 60 days of age, the rats were slow to learn to respond in a shuttle box when a three-tone sequence changed its pattern. Learning to respond when the pitch of a tone was changed one full octave was equal in the experimental and normally reared groups. Again, one of the consequences of sensory deprivation is the reduced ability to integrate a complex stimulus into a readily identified perceptual entity (Riesen, 1972).

Restriction of Tactual-kinesthetic Experience

In 1951 Nissen, Chow and Semmes reported a study of a male chimpanzee whose limbs, including hands and feet, were encased in cardboard mailing tubes from one month to 31 months of age. Fingers, hands and toes could move within the tubes. When the tubes were first removed, standing postures and walking were essentially normal. Guidance of the fingers and their use in poking at objects or picking up food and releasing objects were all done slowly and inaccurately. Strong tactual stimulation produced scratching or withdrawal of the affected limb or body region, but these movements were also slow and inaccurate. Visual guidance was necessary for their execution. With the eyes covered the tactual stimulation produced only a squirming with gross body movement. The chimpanzee also failed in formal training to discriminate two widely separated points of tactual contact. Gradual changes in behavior followed removal of the restriction. There was improvement in grasping, climbing and releasing, but an unusual sitting posture persisted and grooming behavior failed to develop.

Transneuronal Degeneration in the Auditory System

Direct evidence for transneuronal degeneration, having earlier been firmly established for the visual system, was first demonstrated in adult cats following destruction of the cochlea (Powell and Erulkar, 1962). Long survival times are required to permit study of the slow changes that occur in the medial geniculate body. Little visible change in cellular morphology can be seen after only 30 days, but thereafter progressive atrophic effects can be observed with survival times of up to a full year. Between 30 and 60 days after the surgery, the lateral superior olive showed significant shrinkage of the nerve cell diameters. The ventral cochlear nuclei and the medial trapezoid body show similar rates and types of atrophy. A series of studies done not with audition, but with somatosensory pathways, has extended the general finding that transneuronal degeneration occurs much more rapidly in kittens than in adult cats (Riesen, 1966).

Electrophysiology of Binocular Vision After Deprivation

One of the most dramatic changes of function following sensory deprivation that has been found is the loss of binocular cells (Wiesel & Hubel, 1965). Kittens that are prevented from seeing patterns binocularly during a critical period between four and twelve weeks of age are found to have only those units (single cells) of the visual cortex that respond to stimulation of one or the other eye alone. Normally, approximately 90 percent of responsive cells in adult cats respond when either eye is appropriately stimulated, although one eye may be more effective (dominant) than the other. No work of this kind has yet appeared in studies of auditory cells, but there is no good reason to suspect that they will behave differently. A firm answer should shortly be available.

Conclusions

The need for sensory stimulation of the newborn mammalian nervous system if it is to continue its normal growth and differentiation is well documented. While most of the work that does not involve actual surgical destruction has been done with vision, there is ample support for the generality of the principles involved. There is no reason to believe at this time that a critical period during which binaural stimulation is required will not be found for the auditory system.

REFERENCES

Batkin, S., Groth, H., Watson, J.R. and Ansberry, M.: Effects of auditory deprivation on the development of auditory sensitivity in albino rats. *Electroencephalography and Clinical Neurophysiology, 28:*351–359, 1970.

Baxter, B.L.: The effect of visual deprivation during postnatal maturation on the electrocorticogram of the cat. *Experimental Neurology, 14:*224–237, 1966.

Dews, P.B. and Wiesel, T.N.: Consequences of monocular deprivation on visual behavior in kittens. *Journal of Physiology, 206:*437–455, 1970.

Gottlieb, G.: Ontogenesis of sensory function in birds and mammals. In Tobach, E., Aronson, L.R. and Shaw, E. (Eds.): *Biopsychology of Development.* New York: Academic Press, 1971, pp. 67–128.

Nissen, H.W., Chow, K.L. and Semmes, J.: Effects of restricted opportunity for tactual, kinesthetic and manipulative experience on the behavior of a chimpanzee. *American Journal of Psychology, 64:*485–507, 1951.

Powell, T.P.S. and Erulkar, S.D.: Transneuronal cell degeneration in the auditory relay nuclei of the cat. *Journal of Anatomy (London), 96:*249–268, 1962.

Rasch, E., Swift, H., Riesen, A.H. and Chow, K.L.: Altered structure and composition of retinal cells in dark-reared mammals. *Experimental Cell Research, 25:*348–363, 1961.

Riesen, A.H.: Plasticity of behavior: Psychological aspects. In Harlow, H.F. and Woolsey, C.N. (Eds.): *Biological and Biochemical Bases of Behavior.* Madison: University of Wisconsin Press, 1958, pp. 425–450.

Riesen, A.H. Sensory deprivation. *Progress in Physiological Psychology, 1:*117–147, 1966.

Riesen, A.H.: Perceptual entities and forms. *Annals of the New York Academy of Sciences, 193:*150–158, 1972.

Tees, R.C.: Effects of early auditory restriction in the rat on adult pattern discrimination. *Journal of Comparative & Physiological Psychology, 63:*389–393, 1967.

von Noorden, G.K., Dowling, J.E. and Ferguson, D.C.: Experimental amblyopia in monkeys. *Archives of Ophthalmology, 84:*206–214, 1970.

Wiesel, T.N. and Hubel, D.H.: Extent of recovery from the effects of visual deprivation in kittens. *Journal of Neurophysiology, 28:*1060–1072, 1965.

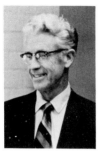

AUSTIN H. RIESEN, Ph.D.

Dr. Riesen was born in Newton, Kansas, and received his A.B. at University of Arizona, Tucson, Arizona, in 1935 and his Ph.D. from Yale University, New Haven, Connecticut, in 1939. He holds a certificate in Aviaiton Physiology from the School of Aviation Medicine. His honors include membership in Phi Kappa Phi; Phi Beta Kappa; Sigma Xi; Fellow, New York Academy of Sciences; Member of International Brain Research Organization, UNESCO; President-elect, 1965–66, President, 1966–67, Division of Physiological and Comparative Psychology, American Psychological Association; American Men of Science; World Who's Who in Science.

Dr. Riesen's wide experiences in the professional and research field include Research Assistant and Assistant Professor, Psychobiology, School of Medicine, Yale University; Aviation Physiology, USAAF; Visiting Research Professor, University of Rochester; Associate Professor, Professor of Psychology, University of Chicago.

Some of the professional organizations to which Dr. Riesen belongs are the American Psychological Association, American Academy of Neurology, American Association for the Advancement of Science, Board of Scientific Advisors, Yerkes Regional Primate Research Center and Consultant, NICHD.

Dr. Riesen has authored numerous articles in scientific and professional journals.

Chapter V

BLINDNESS AND SPATIAL BEHAVIOR*

DAVID H. WARREN

THERE IS A growing realization of the importance of early experience, especially sensory and perceptual experience, for human development. We have already seen good examples of work in this field. Professor Riesen's early research on the primate visual system provided an experimental-comparative basis for much of the more recent work with humans. Dr. White has provided the basis for a vital diagnostic tool: besides knowing what can happen when early perceptual experience is not adequate, it is essential that we have effective diagnostic tools for finding cases early enough for them to be corrected. The work of the HEAR Foundation is an important example of the effectiveness of early remedial intervention in a perceptual disorder. It is this sort of application that is, in fact, the justification for the experimental and the diagnostic efforts.

My own interests are also in the area of early perceptual experience: the thesis that I want to develop has to do with the role of early visual experience in the development of spatial behavior. The questions of space perception have intrigued psychologists for decades and philosophers for centuries. What information do people use in constructing a concept of space and what factors affect their ability to orient and locomote in space? Much of human locomotor behavior, such as picking our way through an obstacle course or walking along a narrow path, is visually guided normally. Much of our closer motor behavior, such as threading a needle, is also visually guided. It is not surprising, therefore, to find that many writers stress the role of vision in structuring the space in which we live.

The apparent dependence of sighted people on vision for their spatial behavior raises specific questions about the spatial behavior of the blind. Are there differences between the congenitally or very early blind and those people who have substantial visual experience and become blind later? What is the effect of the early visual experience? Does it provide a spatial structure that endures after the onset of blindness, or does the adventi-

* A note of thanks is due Linda Anooshian and Janet Bollinger for their help in reviewing the material from which this report is taken.

tiously blind person gradually come to structure his space in the same way that the congenitally blind person must from birth?

One hypothesis about the function of vision for the later blind is that having had vision for some time, the later blind retains a visual frame of reference. Although various writers have approached this notion from different angles, it seems fair to represent the general view as follows. Infants and young children tend to look toward sources of sound, and they tend to track and direct their motor movements, especially hand movements, visually. The result of this accumulated practice in associating spatial events with visual locations is that a visual framework is built up and retained. Then even though the later blind child does not receive any direct visual input, the organizational function of his early visual experience continues to be effective. I want to speak briefly about some research evidence that bears on this general hypothesis about the role of early visual experience.

This work can be treated in several categories. A fairly large part of it deals with motor behavior, including both near-space tasks such as finger maze learning and extended space tasks such as whole-body orientation and locomotion. Another body of research deals with auditory spatial localization and orientation to auditory cues. A third aspect, far less completely studied, has to do with auditory-motor relations and perceptual organization. I will mention representative examples of each type of work.

There have been numerous studies using tactual form discrimination and finger maze learning. I include these types of studies together because they both involve hand performance close to the body. The results of these studies provide a clear indication of the advantage enjoyed by the later blind. An example of such a study is one reported by Worchel (1951). Worchel compared congenitally with adventitiously blind people on several tasks of form recognition and discrimination. In one experiment, he presented the subject with a cutout block and had the subject draw the form, describe it verbally and choose a matching form from a set of four alternatives. In a second experiment, he gave the two parts of a form to the subject's two hands and asked for reports of what the combined form would be. In both these tasks, the adventitiously blind performed better. Furthermore, within the adventitiously blind group, Worchel found a significant positive correlation between performance and the amount of vision that the subject had had before becoming blind. Worchel's study is representative of research with this paradigm: it shows a distinct advantage conferred by early vision.

There has also been a number of studies requiring performance in what could be called *extended space*, as compared to the *near space* tasks that I have just talked about. Worchel (1951) reports such an experiment in the same paper, where he led subjects along one or two sides of a triangle and asked them to walk along a path to complete the right triangle. On this task, Worchel found no differences between the same two groups that had shown differences on the near space tasks. Another example of an extended space task is reported by Cratty (1967). Cratty assessed the so-called *veering tendency* of the blind. Cratty's results are complex, but there are a couple of clear results. Most important, he found that subjects blind from birth veered less than the adventitiously blind. This contradicts the trend from the near space tasks. However, Cratty's group also reports an experiment in which subjects were required to walk along curved paths of varying radius, where the adventitiously blind subjects performed much better than the congenitally blind (Cratty, Peterson, Harris & Schoner, 1968).

Thus when we look at the extended space studies, the pattern of differences is not as clear as for the near space performance. Why should there be this complexity in the pattern of results? Several factors are undoubtedly involved. One such factor may be the length of blind experience. In fact, Cratty's study on veering from a straight line showed that the longer subjects had been blind, the less they veered. Other studies that have looked for correlations between the length of blind experience and performance have typically not found significant relations. I think this ambiguity may be resolved by noting that the length of blind experience factor and the length of early vision factor are not independent. That is, the more early vision a person of a given age has had, the less experience he has had at being blind. The length of early vision factor seems to have a much stronger effect, and on tasks where early vision does confer an advantage, any effect of length of blind experience may be overshadowed. Another factor that is undoubtedly involved is the complexity of the task. It seems to be on the more complex tasks that the length of early vision is important; on the relatively simple tasks such as walking in a straight line, the effect of length of blind experience is allowed to emerge. I'll develop this complexity notion more fully a bit later.

There is much less work on auditory spatial behavior that can be brought to bear on the question of a visual involvement in spatial organization. In the work that has been done, comparisons tend to be made between blind and sighted subjects, with often no differentiation of the early vision characteristics of the blind subjects. Still, some of this work has relevance to our topic. One well-known aspect of the auditory work deals with the phenomenon of facial vision, or obstacle detection, using auditory cues. The blind have often been found to use subtle auditory cues more effectively than blindfolded, sighted subjects, but where practice or training procedures have been used, the sighted subjects have been found to improve very rapidly to the level of performance of the blind (e.g. Supa, Cotzin, and Dallenbach, 1944).

Facial vision really depends on the use of echoes: echodetection and echolocation have also been studied in a sit-down laboratory setting. While these studies have not typically compared the performance of early with late blind, some work reported by Rice and his colleagues is an interesting exception (Rice, Feinstein and Schusterman, 1965; Rice, 1970). Although their numbers of subjects are very small, Rice reports that where differences are found, they favor the early blind both in echodetection and in echolocation. Furthermore, Rice's group has been careful to test their subjects over a longer period of time, and the differences tend to persist.

Several investigators who have undertaken training studies using sound emitters for echo sources have reported very positive results (Kohler, 1964; Juurmaa, 1970). Both blindfolded, sighted subjects and blind subjects improve dramatically, but differences between early and late blind subjects are not routinely reported.

Fisher (1964) reports some extremely interesting work comparing auditory and tactual localization of blind and sighted subjects. The blind subjects were about equal to the sighted subjects at locating simple auditory or tactual targets; however, when they were asked to compare the lateral locations of successively presented auditory and tactual targets, that is, a more complex, cross-model task, the blind were much worse. In a subsequent experiment, Fisher provided the subject with either an auditory or a tactual *reference point* directly before each comparison trial began. The performance of the blind subjects was substantially improved by this procedure, while that of the sighted subjects was not affected very much. It seems possible that the sighted subjects were not aided by this reference point because even with their eyes closed, their visual organization of space continued to provide a very effective reference system within which to compare the auditory and tactual locations. Providing the sighted subjects with a tactual or auditory reference point before each trial did not improve on this visual frame of reference, while even the very simple reference point did improve the performance of the blind, whose spatial organization lacks the visual framework.

While there is little direct evidence about the visual organization of space, the indirect evidence that I have reviewed is largely consonant with the visualization hypothesis. Of the form discrimination, maze performance and body locomotion and orientation work, only the veerying task reported by Cratty (1967) showed a significant superiority of the early blind over the later blind. Of the auditory research, only the echodetection work by Rice (1970) showed an advantage of early blindness. Both of these results are exceptions to the general rule, and both tasks require relatively simple performance. It seems to be on the more complex types of spatial performance that the later blind show a distinct superiority. This may be especially true for tasks requiring people to integrate tactual or motor with auditory information, as in Fisher's work, or to remember one type of information before comparing it with another type.

Early vision, then, may allow the establishment of a frame of reference whose effects endure even after vision is lost. The performance differences between congenitally and adventitiously blind people on the more complex spatial tasks point to the enduring benefit of this frame of reference. Earlier I mentioned a tentative notion about how such a frame of reference might be built up. For auditory spatial information, this may occur through the countless instances of hearing a sound producer, looking, seeing a sound producer and associating the sound location cues with the visual position. There is some recent evidence that even very young infants are sensitive to the correspondence between visual and auditory information: Aronson and Rosenbloom (1971) found that 4- to 8-week-old infants showed distress when their mothers' voices were displaced laterally from their apparent visual positions. It is not difficult to imagine the gradual refinement of this very early tendency to integrate auditory and visual spatial information.

In the case of visual-motor relations, much more is known about the early establishment of cross-modal correspondence. This development may be viewed in various ways: Piaget (1952) speaks of visual and motor schemas, initially independent, which normally become coordinated around three to four months of age. White and Held (1969) describe the infant's progress from the *swiping* stage, around 70 days of age, to mature, visually-directed reaching, around 150 days of age; however the process is described, human infants start off with no visual direction of their motor behavior, and during the first year, they normally acquire a great deal of eye-hand coordination. I suggest that this development may in fact be one of the most important differences between congenitally and adventitiously blind children. If the infant does have vision during the period when his manual activity is emerging, he acquires a basic integration of manual with visual modes. It may be this integration that provides an enduring basis for the more effective use of motor information that seems to characterize the later blind. Thus the first few months of life may indeed be a critical period for the organization of spatial behavior.

There is a second developmental era when the concurrent experience with vision and another function may be especially important. This suggestion is more tentative than the other, and it has to do with the function of language in mediating spatial behavior. Several of the people who have reported the studies on motor behavior have also reported on their subjects' strategies in solving problems such as maze learning and form discrimination (e.g. Knotts and Miles, 1929). In general, they report that subjects who use verbally based strategies are more successful than subjects who use so-called *motor* strategies. It seems reasonable to expect the effectiveness of verbal approaches to be related to the age at onset of blindness. Specifically, if a child lost vision before he had developed his language to the point of labeling the spatial relations that he experienced visually, his later verbal mediation might be less effective than if he had had concurrent verbal behavior and visual experience before becoming blind.

I think this line of reasoning that I've been developing today clearly has some implications for questions of orientation and mobility training for blind individuals, and although I won't have time to more than touch on them, I want to raise some obvious questions. Clearly having had early vision confers certain advantages on the adventitiously blind. However, it may also be that early vision can be a disadvantage. Specifically, dependence on a visual framework may prevent the newly blind person from developing the remaining sensory abilities to their fullest capacity.

This possibility is not merely of casual interest. Should the mobility training of the later blind attempt to maintain and foster the visual frame of reference, or should it discourage reliance on this residual function and encourage strictly non-visual spatial functioning? This question must not be misinterpreted. Many of the perceptual advantages of early vision for the other spatial modalities have already occurred before blinding, and much of the literature indicates that these advantages are not lost with the onset of blindness. The real question is, should the later blind person be encouraged to "think of where you saw this," to encourage his learning to relate new experiences to his residual frame of reference? Or should he be encouraged to experience new stimuli in only those modalities that are now available?

The training question takes a somewhat different form for the congenitally blind. If vision provides an organizational function for the sighted child, and if vision provides a residual organizational framework for the child blinded after two or three years of age, what is the most effective remedial program that can be instituted for the child blind from birth? Certainly mobility programs instituted in the mid-elementary or later years are not optimal, given the apparent importance of early perceptual experience. The fact that only two or three years of early vision can provide a lasting beneficial effect strongly suggests that in normal cases, significant perceptual function becomes established during the first few years. Perhaps spatial perception is especially plastic during that time, but then loses its organizational plasticity. In fact, a great deal of the deprivation research with animals suggests that the period of plasticity may be far less than five years. In short, it seems quite likely that the early years, perhaps up to five, provide the most fertile ground for establishing in the congenitally blind an auditory-motor organization that is maximally useful in structuring spatial relations.

If I have seemed especially concerned with visual function, I want to correct the impression. Although what I've said certainly centers around vision, it really bears on perceptual organization in general, including all sources of information about spatial relations. One dominating theme that is appearing in more and more of our research is the notion that it is an oversimplification to talk about visual perception of space, or auditory or tactual. Space perception may normally be organized around vision, but to be complete, we must speak of all the spatial modalities. A second dominating theme is the importance of early perceptual experience, not just for exercising function, but for establishing and developing function in the first place. This point is illustrated by the role of early vision in spatial behavior, and it is illustrated by the impressive remedial effects of putting hearing aids on very young children.

Finally, I think that the theoretical questions of WHY early experience is so important are far less important than the practical questions. Remedial programs should be structured around the answer to the question: "what works?" We must be receptive to new ideas and to new interpretations of old data. Above all, we must objectively evaluate programs, new and old. We should keep closely oriented to the goal of answering the question: WHAT WORKS?

REFERENCES

Aronson, E. and Rosenbloom, S.: Space perception in early infancy: Perception within a common auditory-visual space. *Science, 172:*1161–1163, 1971.

Cratty, B.J.: The perception of gradient and the veering tendency while walking without vision. *Research Bulletin, American Foundation for the Blind, 14:*31–51, 1967.

Cratty, B.J., Peterson, C., Harris, J. and Schoner, R.: The development of perceptual-motor abilities in blind children and adolescents. *New Outlook for the Blind,* 111–117, 1968.

Fisher, G.H.: Spatial localization by the blind. *American Journal of Psychology,* 77:2–14, 1964.

Juurmaa, J.: On the accuracy of obstacle detection by the blind—Part 2. *New Outlook for the Blind,* 104–118, 1970.

Knotts, J.R. and Miles, W.R.: The maze-learning ability of blind compared with sighted children. *Journal of Genetic Psychology,* 36:21–50, 1929.

Kohler, I.: Orientation by aural clues. *Research Bulletin, American Foundation for the Blind,* 4:14–53, 1964.

Piaget, J.: *The origins of intelligence in children,* 2nd Ed. New York: International University Press, 1952.

Rice, C.E.: Early blindness, early experience, and perceptual enhancement. *Research Bulletin, American Foundation for the Blind,* 22:1–22, 1970.

Rice, C.E., Feinstein, S.H. and Schusterman, R.J.: Echo-detection ability of the blind: Size and distance factors. *Journal of Experimental Psychology,* 70:246–251, 1965.

Supa, M., Cotzin, M. and Dallenbach, K.M.: *Facial vision:* The perception of obstacles by the blind. *American Journal of Psychology,* 57:133–183, 1944.

White, B.L. and Held, R.: Plasticity of sensorimotor development in the human infant. In Rosenblith, J.F. and Allinsmith, W. (Eds.): *Causes of behavior: readings in child development and educational psychology,* 2nd Ed. Boston: Allyn & Bacon, 1969, 60–71.

Worchel, P.: Space perception and orientation in the blind. *Psychological Monographs,* 65:1–28, 1951.

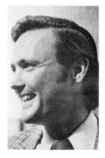

DAVID WARREN, Ph.D.

Dr. Warren received an A.B. in Psychology from Yale College, New Haven, Connecticut, in 1965 and a doctorate from the University of Minnesota, Institute of Child Development in 1969, after which he became Assistant Professor of Psychology at the University of California, Riverside and has served as Acting Chairman, Department of Psychology, (1971–72). In the summer of 1971 he was visiting lecturer, Institute of Child Development, University of Minnesota.

Dr. Warren's research interests center around perception and perceptual development and includes research programs in: Stereoscopic depth perception, visual factors in auditory localization, development of intermodality organization and perceptual factors in reading readiness and achievement. Dr. Warren has had numerous publications in professional journals.

Chapter VI

AUDIOLOGICAL TREATMENT WITH BINAURAL HEARING AIDS

OLE BENTZEN

IN THE INVITATION to this International Conference on Auditory Techniques, the Executive Director of HEAR Foundation, Dr. Ciwa Griffiths, has stated that the science of auditory approach is to teach the deaf child to communicate through the means of an auditory input. When hearing aids are used as a tool to reach the child's brain with clearsound, then intelligible and normal communication will result.

Dr. Griffiths concludes by saying that the HEAR Foundation sponsors this International Conference in the firm belief that the educators of the deaf have a responsibility to explore every avenue possible to improve the role of the deaf in our society.

From a biological, and therefore from a medical, point of view, when treating individuals with reduced hearing from the very start, it is a question of compensating for the defects in the entire acoustic system which are responsible for the reduced ability to hear.

In this connection it is important to bear in mind that the human individual is fitted with one organ of hearing, but with two ears.

The Neuroanatomy of the Organ of Hearing

The peripheral sensory organ of hearing is placed on either side in the right and left cortic organ placed in the cochlea, also called the inner ear. From the environment, the acoustic signals are picked up by the external ear and auditory canal and are led through the ossicles in the middle ear to the sensory organ. Through the first acoustic neuron, the sensory signal is led to the brain-stem-pons, where the greater part of the pathways from the left ear cross the right half of pons, while a lesser number of the pathways run homolateral in pons.

Correspondingly, the pathways from the right hand ear cross over. At the level of the second and third acoustic neurons, some crossing takes place before the sensory signals (after having passed the final synapse, unilaterally through the fourth neuron; acoustic radiation) run up to the acoustic center in the right hand and left temporal lobe.

Both hearing centers thus receive acoustic signals from the right ear as well as the left, though in such a way that the center in the left temporal lobe receives more signals from the right ear, and the center in the right temporal lobe receives more signals from the left ear.

Findings from experimental severing in animals show, however, that left/right representation is poor, since the auditory threshold of both ears is practically unchanged even when the pathways leading to one of the acoustic centers is cut.

On severing the pathways to both centers, we find the animal's ability for frequency-discrimination practically unchanged, but on the other hand, an intensity gain of approximately 70 dB is necessary to obtain the same reaction as before decerebration.

Based on the entire hearing organ's normal neuroanatomy, we can thus establish that the organ of hearing consisting of two peripheral sensory organs, two auditory nerves, three central acoustic neurons and two hearing centers is, for the most part, a single, unmatched organ, especially concerning the representation of the acoustic impulses from the individual's right and left side. Thus it is only the peripheral ear and the auditory nerve, on the right and left sides, respectively, that are dual and designed to catch acoustic impulses from right and left, respectively.

As to localization of defects in the organ of hearing which give rise to chronic hearing loss, results of a large amount of material show that about five percent are localized in the central system, while about 95 percent are localized in the peripheral ear, an estimated 25 percent in the middle ear and 70 percent in the inner ear and auditory nerve.

As it is generally bilateral hearing defects that lead to treatment, it is not possible to give the frequency of one-sided chronic hearing defects.

At a Danish hearing clinic with 4200 patients annually, about 10 percent are found to have asymmetric hearing loss, more than 20 dB difference between the ears.

Why Has Binaural Treatment Not Yet Become Routine?

From our knowledge of the organ of hearing's neuroanatomy and the frequent occurrence of chronic hearing defects in both ears, binaural treatment should, with the present development of modern audiology, be routine treatment to enable optimum acoustic results to be obtained.

The reasons for this not happening are many:

1. The medical audiologists all over the world are primarily educated as otologists, who to a greater degree are trained to direct their diagnosis and

therapy to the peripheral ear, rather than to the unmatched organ of hearing in its entirety.

2. Patients who for years have been plagued with a double sided reduction of hearing probably feel greatly helped when they get a hearing aid for one ear. Through the hearing aid's correction of the frequency perception and through its amplification, they now hear far better—also through the improvement in directional hearing which the use of one hearing aid may give. The hearing aid is still a far from popular means of treatment, and the patients feel that the inconvenience with one aid is more than enough.

3. Hearing aids are in many countries burdened with a large expense for the patient himself as to initial costs, operation and repairs.

By prescribing one hearing aid for a person with a bilateral hearing defect, there is frequent risk of giving him a new handicap. The reasons for this are:

The systematic use of a hearing aid for the right-hand ear, for example, often leads to an unconscious suppression of the left ear's functions—a condition that becomes obvious when transferring to binaural treatment. It may take several years for the patient to learn to use the hearing aid on the left ear.

Systematic use of one hearing aid results in lack of Groen-Hellema effect. (Use of two hearing aids allows 6 dB weaker amplification for both aids than if only one aid is used for one ear.) The one-sided stimulation leads to asymmetrical balance as sound and noise impulses are felt as a cake around the stimulated ear.

Systematic use of one, single hearing aid leads, especially in conversations with two to three people, to a necessary directional forced-head position. The head-worn hearing aid's microphone must be turned towards the speaker. The patient must consider his position in the circle to avoid myoses in neck muscles.

Defective directional hearing, showing as an uncertainty in traffic and great difficulty in following an intermittent conversation among several speakers by lip reading, can also occur. One happens time and time again to miss looking at a speaker because his lack of directional hearing does not warn him in time.

Experiences of Routine Treatment with Binaural Hearing Aids

The Danish system of treating the population with hearing aids is based on an act from 1950. Through public clinics, the hearing aids are distributed without charge to the patients. The hearing aids remain the property of the Invalid Assurance Tribunal, which ensures change of treatment based on doctor's prescription. The 15 audiological clinics in Denmark (population 5.2 million) are all run by medical audiologists; since 1950, there have been treated approximately 130,000 hard-of-hearing and deaf patients.

In the audiological clinic where my experiences originate 4200 patients are treated annually from an area with 780,000 inhabitants. Since 1965, binaural treatment with hearing aids has been routine, as we do not consider a patient with a hearing defect as being sufficiently treated until we have compensated as much as possible for his hearing loss in both the right and left ears.

In the case of nonprescription of binaural hearing aids for persons with bilateral hearing deficiences, the doctors must account for this nonprescription.

To date in this clinic, a total of over 20,000 persons have been treated with binaural hearing aids.

I would like to explain the procedures for treatment of the different grades of hearing deficiencies:

SYMMETRICAL BILATERAL HEARING DEFICIENCY: In the following, the amount of hearing loss is given in TI or TC (Threshold Carhart) measured for the average hearing loss for the frequencies 500, 1000 and 2000 cps. (By asymmetry, it is to be understood the difference in TI or TC for right and left ear is greater than 20 dB.)

In adopting ear-level hearing aids either as ear-hangers or hearing spectacles the necessary conditions were created for placing the hearing aid microphone in the psysiological correct sound-way near the external earcanal.

In the construction of a hearing aid built up with compression which was first used in 1970, the area of use for ear-level hearing aids could be enlarged.

A count of the prescribed treatment for 719 patients, accepted for treatment in October, November and December 1972 shows the following distribution of binaural treatment in relation to the different types of hearing aids, with and without compression:

The treatment of two patients is not shown in Figure VI-1. Both are treated with bilateral hearing spectacles but only with compression in the one side.

It will be seen from the Figure VI-1, that 679 patients (94%) have been prescribed binaural ear-level hearing aids, the relation between hearing spectacles/earhangers being two to three. In 38 percent, hearing aids of the compression type are used.

The total number of patients over the age of 15 years accepted for treatment in October, November and December 1972 is 719 with symmetrical hearing loss, where 385 patients are examined for the first time.

ASYMMETRICAL BILATERAL HEARING DEFICIENCY: In the same three months, 90 patients with asymmetrical hearing loss, *i.e.* difference in TI or TC for right and left ear greater than 20 dB, have been accepted for treatment.

The treatment of one patient is not shown in Figure VI-1. According to the great difference between the hearing loss, this patient has, for the one ear, been prescribed one earhanger and for the other ear, one body

HEARING LOSS IN DECIBEL					
	0–30	31–60	61–80	over 81	total
Number	143	491	68	17	719
Percent	20	68	10	2	

BINAURAL HEARING AID TREATMENT			
Model:	total		percent
Body aids	38		6
Ear-hangers	232	390	54
Ear-hangers plus compr.	158		
Hearing spectacles	174		
Hearing spectacles plus compr.	102	289	40
Hearing spectacles bone-conduction	13		
Total:	717		

Figure VI-1

aid. It will be seen from the Figure VI-2 that 82 patients (92%) have been prescribed ear-level hearing aids, half with hearing spectacles and half with earhanger. In only eight percent hearing aids of the compression type are used.

From the total of 90 patients, 47 are treated for the first time. The difference in the hearing loss between the good and the bad ear is shown in Figure VI-2. About 30 percent of the patients have a difference greater than 40 dB. This problem has especially been focused, as some therapists have the opinion that a too great a difference between the hearing loss makes binaural hearing aid treatment impossible. This is not the experience in our work.

From Figure VI-2 it is seen that 23 patients have a very slight hearing loss in the best ear, *i.e.* 30 dB or less. Even these are prescribed binaural hearing aids as a consequence of an investigation showing good results by open-mould technic in patients with very steep curve in the audiogram.

Experiences of Routine Treatment with Binaural Hearing Aids in Children

Deaf and hard-of-hearing children up to the age of 15 years have, in this clinic, been systematically treated with binaural hearing aids since 1956.

Serious cases of bilateral loss of hearing have always indicated treatment

HEARING LOSS IN DECIBEL—BEST EAR

	20	25	30	35	40	45	50	55	60	65	70	total
Number	5	8	10	14	16	10	8	7	4	5	3	90
Diff. in dB between the ears		23	24	13	9	8	6	5	2	1	0	

HEARING AID TREATMENT

Model	monaural	binaural		percent
Body aids		7		8
Ear-hangers		35	49	48
Ear-hangers plus compr.		7		
Hearing spectacles		28		
Hearing spectacles plus compr.	1	8	40	44
Hearing spectacles bone-conduction		3		
Total			89	

Figure VI-2. Treatment with hearing aids of 90 patients with asymmetrical hearing loss.

with body-aid, either as a single aid with a V-cord and telephone in the right and left ear. In this way, it has been ensured that the child, in the case of trouble with a defective aid, always has amplification for at least one ear.

The principal, motivation has been to get the child examined as early as possible and to treat it on suspicion of hearing loss. The children in treatment with hearing aids are kept under guidance of a teacher of the deaf or by the district nurse, who makes visits to the home. The children are placed in ordinary nursery schools from the age of three, in order to secure optimal development of language in the deaf child through constant exposure to normal speech and language from its classmates in the nursery school. This treatment has, since its start in 1952, shown how modern audiological treatment of deaf children is able to place the child in the centers for special education in the ordinary school. Deaf children without this audiological rehabilitation had to be placed in former times at the school for the deaf.

The children under audiological treatment are called for control at the audiological clinic at least once every year.

A count of the prescribed treatment for 50 children accepted for treat-

HEARING AID TREATMENT OF PERCEPTIVE DEAFNESS IN CHILDREN

AGE	1	2	3–4	5–6	7–15	total
number	4	5	10	8	23	50
first exam.	4	1	3	2	2	12

HEARING TI dB	0-30	31-60	61-80	over 80	OBS	
number	8	20	8	11	3	50
first exam.	1	5	1	2	3	12

HEARING AID TREATMENT

Model	Symm.	Asymm.
Body aid V-cord	9 (4)	
Body aid x 2	9 (2)	1
Phonic ear V-cord	2	
Earhanger x 1	4 (1)	6 (2)
Earhanger x 2	22 (2)	2
Earhanger over cross		3
Hearing spectacles x 2	1	
No aid	3 (3)	2 (2)
Total	50 (12)	14 (4)

Figure VI-3. Treatment with hearing aids of 50 children with symmetrical and asymmetrical hearing loss caused by perceptive deafness.

ment in October, November and December 1972 shows the following distribution of treatment:

It will be seen from the Figure VI-3 that 50 patients of the 64 children had symmetrical perceptive hearing defect. Twelve patients among these have been examined for the first time.

Twenty children in this group have been treated with body-aids (40%), half with one body-aid and V-cord and half with two body-aids. Since 1972, we have introduced the special body-aid Phonic Ear, which consists of two interconnected aids and has, thanks to its construction with compression, proved to be greatly superior to the ordinary body-aids in children with extreme hearing loss.

Among the 14 children with asymmetrical hearing loss greater than 20 dB, nearly all have been treated with ear-level hearing aids. Even as we have been able to use hearing spectacles in children down to the age of 8 years of age, the earhangers are the routine treatment in children at this age.

BINAURAL HEARING AID TREATMENT
PATIENTS

| | | | MODEL OF HEARING AIDS | | |
	No.	percent	BODY AID	EAR HANGER	HEARING SPECTACLES
AGE		%	%	%	%
15–59	80	21	3	41	56
60–79	234	61	4	51	48
over 80 years	71	18	4	85	11
HEARING					
LOSS in dB		%	%	%	%
0–30	113	30	0	44	56
31–60	264	68	1	65	34
61–79	7	2	six	one	
over 80 dB	1		one		
Total No.	385		10	215	160
percent			3	56	41

Figure VI-4. Treatment with binaural hearing aid in 385 adults in relation to age and to hearing loss.

The Model of Hearing Aids Used in Binaural Treatment

Binaural hearing aid treatment can be established either with body-aids or with ear-level hearing aids. The last model, either as ear-hangers or hearing spectacles, are the only ones which will give the patient the opportunity to establish a better directional hearing.

The distribution of the different models of hearing aids used in binaural treatment is seen in Figure VI-4, which represents 385 adults with symmetrically hearing loss.

In only 3 percent, body-aids have been used. For ear-level hearing aid, the use of hearing spectacles decreases with increasing age. Among 71 patients over the age of 80 years, about 10 percent were prescribed hearing spectacles, whereas 85 percent received ear-hangers.

The use of hearing spectacles also decreases with increasing hearing loss. Among 264 patients with a hearing loss between 31 and 60 dB, one-third were prescribed hearing spectacles and two-thirds ear-hangers. Eight patients had a hearing loss greater than 61 dB, and all were prescribed body-aids.

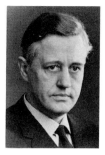

OLE BENTZEN, M.D.

Dr. Bentzen was born in Denmark. He received his medical degree in 1943. Since 1951, Dr. Bentzen has received outstanding recognition as a specialist in the field of otology serving as the director of the State Hearing Center, Aarhus, Denmark since 1952. In 1962 Dr. Bentzen became Assistant Professor in Audiology at the University of Aarhus and was appointed consultant for the World Health Organization, European offices. At present Dr. Bentzen is the Audiological Consultant for Danida a position to which he was appointed by the Danish foreign ministry in 1967.

Chapter VII

INTEGRATION: PURPOSE AND PRACTICE

Lois E. Tarkanian

THE CONCEPT of the *open classroom* in elementary education has emerged during the last eight to ten years. Along with this open movement, increased emphasis is being placed upon the social and psychological benefits accrued from educating handicapped children in regular classroom settings. Educators in general, as well as those in special education, are aware of the importance of the natural language environment and the psychological implications of maintaining social integrity.

The recent emphasis on noncategorical educational programs for exceptional children, however, has created a number of problems for educators. Most would endorse the philosophy that exceptional children should be maintained in regular classes whenever possible and that the use of labels should be de-emphasized, but difficulties are being met as we attempt to translate this philosophy into a practical and valid program.

I am not going to linger today on the logistics of the problem. That is, who should integrate and when and in what subject area. As we at Oralingua have moved more fully into the mainstream of cooperative class placement, we have found these areas have caused the least amount of difficulty.

Because of our role as a small, private school, our integration program at Oralingua has developed into four different steps.

Step I is a placement in self-contained deaf classes. All new pupils to the program are placed in self-contained classes until our personnel have an opportunity to know the child, assess how he learns, thinks, reacts. We must know to some extent what a child's strengths and weaknesses are before integration occurs.

Step II is placement in a combined hearing and deaf class on the Oralingua campus. This provides for us a more effective, economical use of personnel as integration begins. Our staff has a closer guidance over curriculum, content and direction. At this level, we learn a great deal about how the deaf child interacts with hearing peers in an educational setting, and we can assist and guide parents in the areas in which the child needs help.

Step III consists of placement of pupils into public and private hearing schools within a five-mile radius of Oralingua. An Oralingua staff member, Miss Geraldine Porter, coordinates this aspect of the program. She spends approximately one full morning every school day within the hearing classes, observing deaf pupils, providing supportive tutoring, providing inservice training for teachers and maintaining appropriate administrative contacts. The deaf pupils return in the afternoon for additional work at Oralingua. Each deaf pupil receives individual tutoring daily, as well as assistance in group activities where needed. A great amount of concentration is spent on this and the previous level in helping the deaf pupil learn how to attend well when working within a group and learning how to follow directions given to a group.

Step IV is placement in hearing classrooms within local schools within a family's neighborhood. This involves full-day placement in a school near where the child lives, where siblings, if any, and friends also attend. The deaf child receives one full morning and one full afternoon each week of supportive assistance from an Oralingua teacher. This includes observation of the deaf child within the classroom environment, tutoring of the pupil in appropriate areas, counseling with teacher and with parents and public relations work with personnel in neighborhood school. The tutor from Oralingua and the classroom teacher work closely together. For example, covering the definitions of "nose," "nosey" and "knows" may be difficult for the deaf child or "just the same," "just a minute" or "just alike." The classroom teacher has too many children within her class to spend a disproportionate amount of time with one, yet the deaf child does need extra assistance. The tutor can spend the extra time needed. We have found the reading textbooks abound with idioms, and additional help is definitely needed there. Surprisingly, when work was done on phonics such as vowel sounds 'a' and 'e' in recognition in words such as 'pat' and 'pet,' our deaf pupils have done very well. Placement with hearing peers within their own neighborhood school has made them feel more socially relaxed. They seem to have better motivation for higher levels in speech and language. They have not been reluctant to talk in front of the class, to use language in socialization, and they have shown, in most cases, a high degree of independence.

Although, for the purpose of this presentation, these steps are clearly designated into a four-step structure, in practice the steps interblend, and there is a great amount of flexibility so that a child may be placed and moved according to his specific individual needs.

Some of the skills upon which we concentrate with children in Steps II and III in preparation for Step IV are:

1. *Ability to follow directions for seatwork.* Instructions are not usually repeated more than once or twice by classroom teacher. After directions have been given, the teacher of the deaf often asks a child to repeat back what he is going to do, to make sure he understands correctly. If he does not, she reviews instructions and attempts to determine where he missed out and what help he needs.

2. *Ability to follow oral discussion in small group.* Optimum use of residual hearing is very important here. It takes patience on the part of all for a child to learn who is speaking when.

3. *Ability to follow oral reading in a group.*

4. *Ability to work independently,* to complete tasks without being reminded or receiving any further directions from the teacher.

5. *Ability to use "free time" wisely.*

6. *Ability to know when one doesn't understand* either directions, questions or assignment and to tell the teacher about the misunderstanding. This is the most difficult area of need.

If your deaf program has a solid curriculum with a dedicated, well-trained staff, it will not be difficult to know when a child is ready for intergration. Oralingua gives three different academic achievement tests to pupils as this assessment is occurring. These tests are the Wide Range Achievements, the Stanford Achievement and the California Achievement Tests. With scores from three different tests, we are able to determine quite accurately the academic functioning of the child. Language assessment is conducted on the Utah Test of Language Development, as well as through assessment of video tape samples. Social adjustment is determined through some psychological testing, but primarily upon staff judgment.

Social and psychological implications are stressed when integration occurs, but we do not underestimate the importance of academics. Let's face it, it is the academics which are stressed in the majority of hearing schools today. Academics and social behavior are the yardsticks usually used in judging pupils within our public schools. If we are after true, full integration of our deaf pupils, not tokenism, then we should expect our deaf children to perform well, academically and socially, within the normal limits of the regular classroom. That is, if a deaf child has above-average academic potential, then we should not expect and accept average performance as he participates with his hearing peers in the regular classroom.

We realize, of course, that the child is always going to need backup work if this goal is to be obtained. He is deaf today, will be deaf tomorrow, next week and years to come unless additional major medical advancements are made. The deafness is there, so strong supportive follow-up work will be needed. And we tell parents whose children are being integrated into hearing schools: "Don't relax now. Some of you think you've made it and can work less with your child. Don't kid yourself. You will need to work even harder. You will be within an educational environment whose major interest is not deafness. You will be with teachers inundated with the details of working with 25 to 36 pupils, not just six or seven. You often will be working with attitudes untouched by recent advances in educating deaf children. A parent of a hearing child can slip a little, sluff off once in a while and then catch up and make up for what is lost. You cannot. Your child is deaf and no matter how well he functions now, if you want that comparative level maintained, you do not let up one bit."

We are finding the major problems of integration exist *not within* the deaf child, but within the *attitudes* and the *curriculum content* present in the classroom into which the child is integrating. No matter what care we take, no matter how much time we spend, no matter how much effort is expended in selection of cooperative classroom personnel, we still find significant problems to overcome. In talking with Winifred Northcott during the break, I found she, too, was concerned with this area and had made application for a grant for inservice training for teachers who would have deaf pupils in their classrooms. With a concentrated effort like that, perhaps, a change in attitudes can be made.

Let me now show you a video clip of a child preparing to enter Step IV of our integration program. We do not own a port-a-pak at our school and could not film within his current placement in a regular classroom, but we can show you his performance prior to his enrolling in a public school in his neighborhood. We will view him in a listening skill activity in chart story work. Please note his audiogram on the overhead. He definitely falls within the definition of deaf, yet you will see him utilize listening skills on a hard-of-hearing level. The chart story with which he is working was written following a class study trip to the mountains. Within this clip you will see the teacher eventually give him four complex sentences auditorially. (Show video tape clip of severely deaf child, age 7.)

This child has excellent listening skills. On familiar subjects, he perceives on audition alone. We have found that on the introduction of new, unfamiliar, more complex material, he performs better if he utilizes lipreading along with the audition.

Now keep in mind that child. He is similar to other pupils integrating into hearing classes. Keep him in mind and think of these comments:

Poor child; he's deaf. I had a deaf child in my class once eight years ago. He couldn't understand a thing, had to be placed in a special class. Why don't you have this child go into a special class? Poor little kid, he needs to be with his own.

If you really want deaf children to be independent, don't give them extra help. He could do those problems if he wants to. Does he understand the directions? Of course, he does. I asked him and he said yes.

How will he understand me? I don't know signs.

I worry about his fibbing. My roommate read that most deaf people are paranoid. I don't know.

We're so lucky the people on yard duty are aware he is deaf. Remember how he got hit on the head with that ball because he was deaf. Oh, your other son gets hit on the head with balls on the playground and he's not deaf. Well . . .

He's not deaf. How could he be? He can hear almost everything I say even if he can't see me.

Can he talk?

After seeing the video clip of this child—his speech, language, ability to follow directions, ask questions, to listen—these questions don't seem very appropriate do they? And yet these are comments I have heard over the past twelve months pertaining to pupils intergrating into hearing classrooms yet functioning similarly to what you saw on the video clip. It behooves each of us to extend a maximum effort to redirect many of the attitudes prevelant today about deaf individuals.

Keep in mind this child and think of this pertaining to his curriculum:

Two years ago he was studying the urban, suburban communities, developing concepts about the interdependence of people, some producing goods, some providing services. He visited factories, assembly lines, and he role-played what he saw.

One year ago this child was studying the varying geographical locations in California. He was developing concepts about the interdependence of farm and mountain areas and ocean and desert areas. He was able to spontaneously discuss the similarities between a mountain village and a city, i.e. both have electricity, both have workers.

This year the class he was in is studying early California and developing concepts concerning the interdependence between the Indians and their environment; they are comparing the illiterate tribes of today (i.e. Tassadays in Phillipines and Masai of Kenya with the California Indians). They are studying the cultural impact on environments by moving into the Spanish settlers and their effect on California.

From this type of social science background, we have pupils in hearing classes taking turns reading from a book about children in other lands or spending perhaps a total of four hours listening to the teacher read about another land. From a concept-, experience-oriented curriculum to a fact-, memorization-oriented curriculum, these children have moved. Each of us must also work towards curriculum improvement in all types of classes, and, in the meantime, we must give our deaf children skills that will allow them to get a handle on what will occur within most regular classrooms without losing too much of concepts already laid.

Attitudes within the children are most important as integration begins. We work upon:

1. wanting to be the center of attention
2. moving from adult-child interaction to child-child interaction
3. developing a feeling of confidence.

We will now see a video tape section of children ready for Step III as they interact within a group. Our social science and science programs are our major vehicles for this type of social and verbal interaction. (Show video tape of class of 6 pupils discussing rules of behavior while having a picnic at the park.)

I have here a few examples of the four integration steps of our program:

Step I

Video tape showing profoundly deaf children new to Oralingua enrolled in self-contained deaf class.

Step II

Video tape showing deaf and hearing children intermingling in classroom on Oralingua campus during singing, describing objects and free option time.

Step III

Video tape showing hearing and deaf children interacting in class activities at Broad Oaks Nursery School on Whittier College campus.

You've already seen preliminary preparation to *Step IV* on the first video tape clip presented of a seven-year-old child working on chart-story listening skill activity.

I hope the information and video tapes presented here today will be of some assistance in adding additional information towards the betterment of integration for deaf pupils.

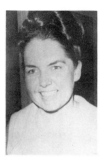

LOIS E. TARKANIAN, M.A.

Mrs. Tarkanian received her B.A. in general elementary education and her M.A. in speech and hearing at Fresno State University. She holds California State credentials in administration, general elementary, speech and hearing and deaf education, as well as clinical certification in Speech Pathology and Audiology from the American Speech and Hearing Association. Her experience includes teaching and administration in regular classes in elementary schools; aphasic, deaf and hard-of-hearing classes; speech pathologist with voice, language and speech problems. Mrs. Tarkanian has held chairmanships and offices in California Speech and Hearing Association; American Speech and Hearing Association; Inland Empire Speech and Hearing Association. She is also a member of California Assocation of Teachers of Deaf and Hard of Hearing Children; California Association of Parents of Deaf and Hard-of-Hearing Children; Council for Exceptional Children; Alexander Graham Bell Association; Conference of American Instructors of the Deaf and has served as consultant in curriculum, deaf education and speech and hearing for various districts in California.

She is currently Administrator of Oralingua School for Hearing-Impaired Children. Previously she was Consultant in Speech and Hearing for San Bernardino County Schools.

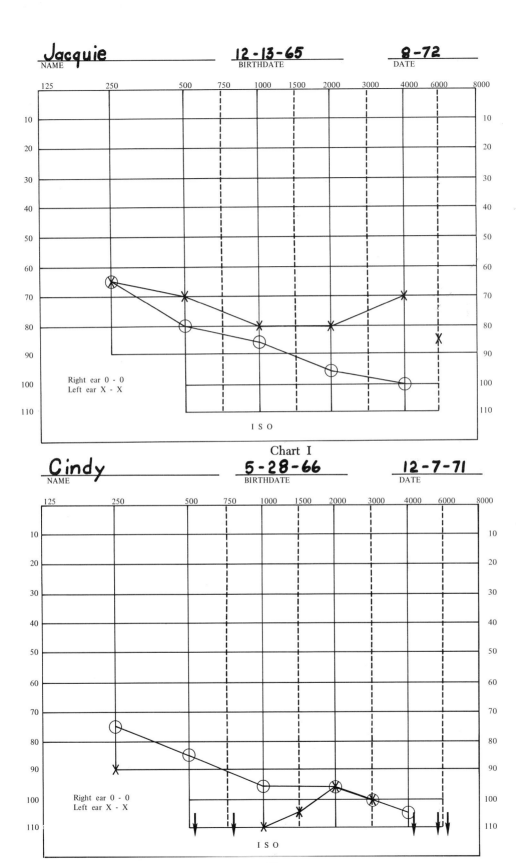

Chart I

Chart II

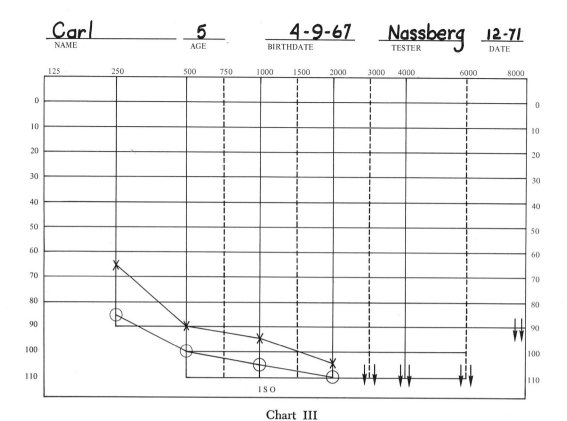

Chart III

Leigh Anne   5   12-25-66   E. Turner   3-73
NAME   AGE   BIRTHDATE   TESTER   DATE

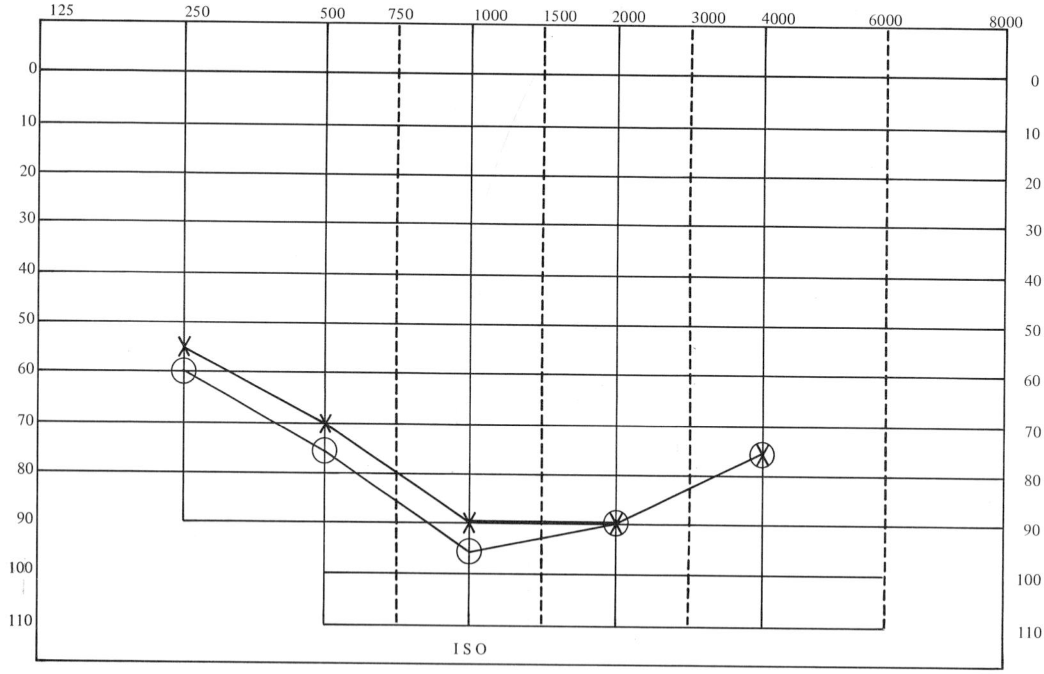

Chart IV

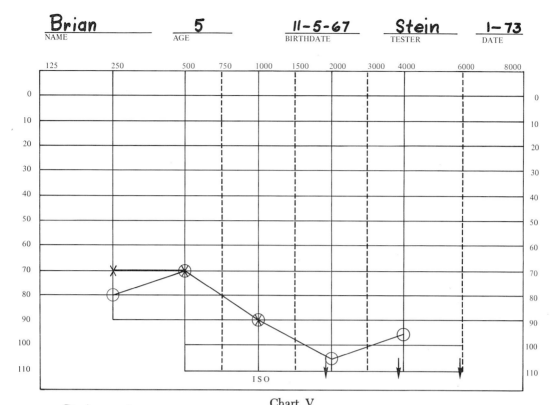

NAME: Brian AGE: 5 BIRTHDATE: 11-5-67 TESTER: Stein DATE: 1—73

Chart V

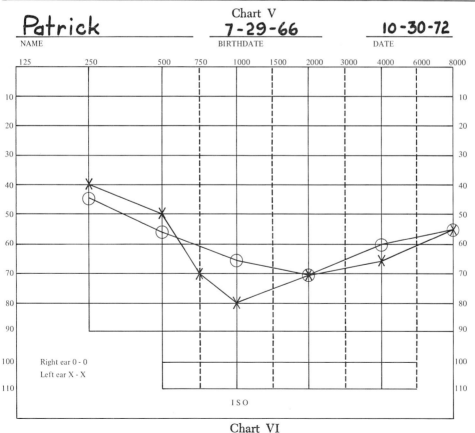

NAME: Patrick BIRTHDATE: 7-29-66 DATE: 10-30-72

Right ear 0 - 0
Left ear X - X

ISO

Chart VI

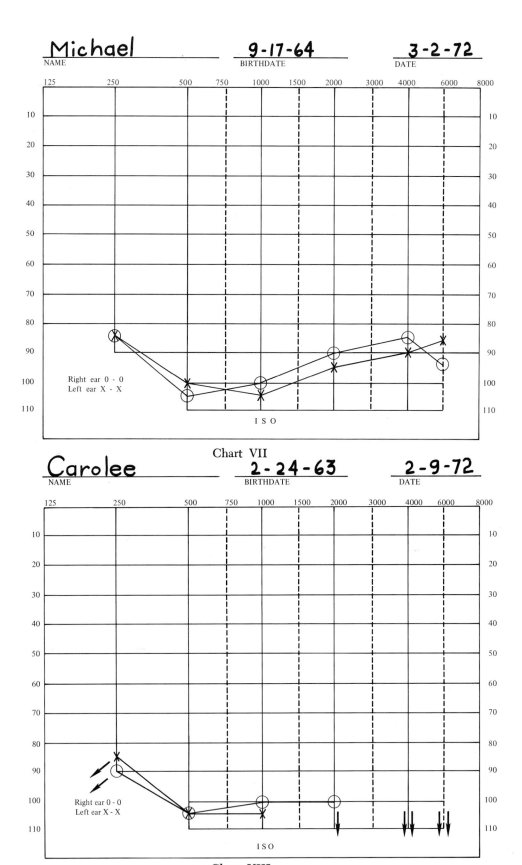

Chart VII

Chart VIII

Chapter VIII

AGAINST THE CURRENT

PRISCILLA PITTENGER MUIR

EDUCATIONAL PHILOSOPHY, policy and procedure seem to function like tides, always moving, never still. The currents push relentlessly in one direction and then reverse and move quite inexorably in the other. One must either go with the tide of the moment or swim as strongly as possible against the current. At the present time in the education of children with severe hearing impairment, the tide has become a veritable tidal wave threatening to engulf all persons in its path—children, parents, educators, audiologists and other concerned persons. This tidal wave has a name—*total communication*. Persons who believe in the oral education of deaf children must swim against the strong current of this wave.

Remember that if one is to swim against a strong-running current, one has no time to look for sharks or to dodge debris. Accordingly, I shall not discuss the validity of research which has ridden the crest of the wave; I shall not discuss whether *total communication* is what it purports to be, though I believe it seldom is, and I shall not discuss the children for whom manual communication may be indicated. I do propose to discuss reasons for strong swimmers to keep their courage and determine at least to stay afloat. In fact, the swimmers must look for beachheads.

To borrow a term from N.A.S.A., all systems are *go* at this time for the most efficient oral instruction ever available to deaf children. Advances in technology, especially in electronics and acoustics, growth of information concerning how children learn and the development of the sciences of linguistics and psycholinguistics have combined to provide new dimensions for the always difficult task of compensating for severe deafness. None of these systems is being adequately used in most schools for the deaf, and it is perhaps necessary to examine reasons for our failure to capitalize on what is available. If we see those reasons clearly, we can perhaps reach for the handholds which will help us to swim against the current.

A quarter of a century ago at the New York Regional Office of the Veterans Administration, I saw some very deaf men put together limited cues and manage to understand sentences through audition alone. In 1948 a hearing aid had only a limited range and provided no more than 35-decibels gain. I raised the question whether deaf children should not be able to learn to use minimal residual hearing and to comprehend speech as the men were doing. I was told unequivocally that they could not, that the men could do it because they already knew sound and language and could synthesize from minor cues, but that no child could be expected to develop use of similar residual hearing to the point of learning through his ears. I still thought perhaps children could. Several years were to pass before Ciwa Griffiths and I got together, and I was to hear someone else state a conviction that young deaf children could learn to use their hearing functionally. In the years since the HEAR Foundation began to examine this hypothesis, many clinics have come to agree with the basic premise. It is nevertheless true that, in general, the residual hearing of children is quite inadequately explored.

Why is this still true in 1973? There are several reasons. First: many people of influence in the education of the deaf simply do not believe that amplification can do much for very deaf children. Some of the most vocal people in this group are members of the adult deaf society, many of them born deaf or deafened long before there was amplification which could help them. Others are individuals of integrity who have not seen it happen and therefore believe it can't.

Second: there has been an almost unbelievable lack of communication between the disciplines most concerned with deaf children, the audiologists and the teachers. Because this is true, children have often had too much or too little amplification or otherwise inappropriate hearing aids, the exploration of the child's potential has not been carried forward, hearing aids have been inadequately maintained and the on-going emphasis on listening has been minimal.

Third: too little information has been given to manufacturers of auditory aids. The aids which congenitally deaf children need are not necessarily those which are presently available. Obviously manufacturers are in business and are concerned about producing instruments which people will purchase and use consistently. They require specific information and suggestions before they turn their attention to new design.

Fourth: for many years, the only amplification to which most deaf children were exposed was the classroom, group hearing aid. Children with all types and degrees of deafness receive essentially the same amplification on a group aid though they can, of course, control the volume to some degree. If the unit needs repair, *all* of the children are without amplification. Teachers are accustomed to group aids and tend to be quite uncritical of their performance, many believe that high fidelity, strong signal is necessary for initial exposure to sound. Manufacturers and sales-men vigorously promote them, and group aids of several kinds are still in wide use. Too little research is available to provide clear information on their desirability, but at this time it seems necessary to examine the alternative of individual, wearable aids.

Fifth: most teachers simply do not know enough about amplification nor about developing listening habits and skills. To tell the truth, I think most audiologists don't either. Since I have been in teacher education a long time, I regret making this admission.

One of the beachheads toward which we must swim at this time is improved use of amplification. This implies strong ties between the class-room and the clinic with accurate exchange of information in a climate of mutual respect. It implies making suggestions to manufacturers because the technical competence is now available to produce what is needed. It implies working consistently on a child's ability to listen and compre-hend. Perhaps most of all, it implies an optimistic, believing attitude which recognizes that some hearing is surely available and should be used.

We turn now to information about children's learning. How psychology has changed since my first course in it! Forty-five years ago I was taught that children learned basically through repetition until neurological con-nections to the brain were fixed. In the years since that theory was dominant, many changes have taken place, and much research has been conducted into how children learn. A wide variety of thinking processes has been examined, and the progression in which children normally learn those processes is emerging. Teachers have always been adjured to require children to think, but only in recent years have analyses been made which define thinking tasks. At this time teaching children to think has many components and opens many avenues to exploration.

We used to be told that a deaf child entering school was a *blank page* because he had no verbal language. At that time children entered school at five or six; now they come at three or younger. No child can live a thousand days (the three-year-old) without learning a great deal about the world in which he lives. How he uses the information which he has acquired through observation and experience is the substance of his cog-nitive growth. It can be held to a primitive level or developed into sophis-ticated thinking both nonverbally and verbally.

Deaf children have long been spoon fed almost all of their learning. They were always taught two operations and sometimes not much more, i.e to match and to memorize. From their first days in school, they matched words to objects and ideas, and in later years they matched answers to questions. They memorized words, forms, rules and information but ma-nipulated ideas very sparingly. They were told exactly what to do in every activity, and in general they sought the one and only acceptable answer to every situation.

Making use of the psychology of our day and recognizing the considerable information in the child's possession, the teacher can encourage him in many kinds of thinking. Let us look at a couple of examples. Suppose that the teacher has brought to school an ordinary kitchen strainer. To encourage divergent thinking, the children are asked how that strainer might be used in the classroom. (Recently my college class suggested twenty-eight different ways that a strainer might be used, many of which would probably occur to children, even very little children. Children might also propose what would not occur to an adult.) Observe that conveying their suggestions requires *language*. To encourage problem solving, the strainer might be one of several tools which the *children* would propose as means of cleaning the fishbowl.

The deaf child, like any other small human being, has the capacity to think. As we explore the kinds of thinking that children normally do, we find that the hearing-impaired child can use his brains in the same ways. What he requires is the challenge and the opportunity. As he learns to think, he will also need to talk. The cognitive processes are another beachhead toward which our strong swimmers must head if they are to escape the tidal wave.

Next, we need to look at linguistics and psycholinguistics. Thoroughly entrenched in the area of education of the deaf is the notion of grammar-based acquisition of language. The modern linguist tells us that the grammar we learned has its origin in Latin and is often not applicable to English. Many new forms of grammar are emerging; patterning, transformational grammar, tagmemics, etc. Even if we continue to work on a grammar base, there are new possibilities for more flexible language learning and of course more flexible language usage. Linguistics is a relatively new science, and one has only to read some of its literature to know that it is still experimental and lacks cohesion, but much research is being carried forward which must come to have an impact on educating hearing-impaired children. Psycholinguistics, too, is exploring language development. From this discipline we learn that children's syntax is different from adult syntax and that there are progressive steps in children's acquisition of their native languages. The application of psycholinguistic principles will surely lead us to some changes in our traditional procedures. First: a much longer period of input will be allowed before children are expected to respond verbally. Second: attention to intonation patterns will be stressed. Third: performance expected from the child will be much less exact, and correction will be casual rather than insistent. Fourth: language exposure will be greatly increased, much more vocabulary and greater variety of language forms will be used by teachers and parents.

Fifth: teachers will become much more aware of the child's emerging syntax, less concerned about its initial accuracy and better equipped to build on it and expand it. These two disciplines, linguistics and psycholinguistics, are another beachhead which must be reached.

For more than fifty years, I have been surrounded by the problems of educating deaf children. This is a professional field which has always had great autonomy and which has insisted upon unbelievable isolationism. It has created its own authorities and listened only to them. At convention after convention, the same speakers are heard (I was one of those speakers for many years, and I'm quite sure I didn't have *that* much to say.) Sorely needed now is an infusion of fresh plasma. I think that infusion should come from two sources: individuals from other fields than our own and experimental classroom teachers who are working with children every day. Most of us who rise to speak have not taught children for a long, long time.

In closing, I want to ennunciate my personal credo:

I believe in deaf children, their capabilities and their potential.

I believe in the good will of persons who work with the children but believe they need new techniques.

I believe that speech is the inalienable right of the human being and every effort must be made to help the deaf child acquire oral competence.

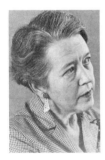

PRISCILLA PITTENGER MUIR, Ed.D.

A.B. from Indiana University in 1929; M.A. from Teachers College at Columbus, Ohio, in 1941; Ed.D. from Stanford University at Palo Alto, California in 1955.

Priscilla Pittenger Muir, daughter of Oscar M. Pittenger, Superintendent of Indiana Schools for the Deaf grew up at the Institute and received her original preparation in the training classes there. She taught for ten years in the Alexander Graham Bell Day School for the Deaf in Cleveland, Ohio. She served two years in the U.S. Navy as a WAVE, one of these years in Aural Rehabilitation at the U.S. Naval Hospital in Philadelphia, Pa. For two years she worked in rehabilitation at the New York Regional Office of the Veterans Association; she also taught one year in the Ohio State School for the Deaf before coming to California State University at San Francisco where she has directed the program preparing teachers of the deaf from 1949 to date.

Chapter IX

CRITICAL AGE IN HEARING

JUDITH B. EBBIN

THE MOTIVATION for this paper arose partly out of some intriquing clinical findings consistently observed for nearly two decades by the HEAR Foundation and partly out of my own long-standing interest in the concept of critical age. Appropriate to a discussion of critical periods is the timing of this International Conference, for at this point in time, on an interdisciplinary basis, we have entered a most critical era in terms of auditory techniques.

Just as the impetus and supporting structure for the auditory approach has been derived from developmental psychology, educational psychology, etc., and not from a traditional education of the deaf basis, the supporting structure which merges hearing impairments and critical age is similarly not to be found in the deaf education literature—yet. The evidence for the ideas which shall be elaborated comes from experimental psychology, developmental psychology and neurophysiological bases.

Communication disorders, particularly when approached from a multi-disciplinary orientation, offer a supreme opportunity to examine temporal relationship ramifications of diagnosis and therapeutic intervention. The Identification/Intervention Quotient, a hypothetical quantitative classification system one might use to analyze time factors, varies according to the nature of each disorder. Thus, the aggressiveness in initiating therapy for a four-year-old child with articulation problems involving the /r/ and /s/ sounds, for example, differs drastically from the urgency with which therapy for hearing impairments is currently initiated by many of us. Figure IX-1 illustrates the Identification/Intervention Quotient with examples of its hypothetical use.

If one did use such a ratio to highlight the differences with which various communication disorders are subjected to therapy, the more closely the ratio approximated 1.00, the more urgent the need to initiate therapy. Determining age at suggested intervention is derived from clinical experience by many of us and reinforced by theories of early childhood development. Inherent in the auditory approach, stressing early detection

Figure IX-1
IDENTIFICATION/INTERVENTION QUOTIENT

$$\frac{\text{Age at identification}}{\text{Age at suggested intervention}} \quad \text{equals an urgency indicator}$$

Example: articulation problem

$$\frac{\text{age at identification: 4 years}}{\text{age at intervention: 6 years}} \quad = \quad .67$$

Example: hearing impairment

$$\frac{\text{age at identification: 3 months}}{\text{age at intervention: 3 months}} \quad = \quad 1.00$$

and early therapeutic intervention, is a philosophy which synthesizes key factors in the complex process of human development. One classification scheme of psychological concepts pertaining to developing human potential might be the following, as indicated in Figure IX-2. Two most important notions embedded in the classification scheme derive from re-

Figure IX-2
CLASSIFICATION SCHEME OF PSYCHOLOGICAL CONCEPTS PERTAINING TO DEVELOPMENT

Psychological Concept	Definition	Change Agent
Growth	Typically denotes increases in size— height, weight and muscle size, for example	Used to be considered entirely genetic; now known that influence of environmental factors is considerable.
Maturation	Linear growth and emergence of specific capacities.*	Interaction between genetic and environmental factors.
Learning	Changes in behavior not simply ascribable to growth processes.**	Interaction between genetic and environmental factors—involves growth and maturation.
Development	A general term to denote totality of full blossoming and multiple uses of emerging functions and skills.*	Interaction between genetic and environmental factors—involves growth, maturation and learning.

*Lewis,   1971.
**Ragan and Shepherd, 1971.

search findings indicating manipulable aspects of genetic versus environmental interaction. These notions are critical period and sensory deprivation.

Critical period refers to a stage in development during which certain structures or capacities are irreversibly formed at a specific time and not at any other time. A modification of the irreversibility aspect of critical period is the concept of *sensitive period*, which states that at certain times an individual can learn some things more efficiently, more quickly or with less training than at other times. The philosophy of early identification/early intervention has been couched in terms of the sensitive period notion.

Freedman (1961) cites types of experimental situations in which sensory deprivation has been studied:

1) that in which the attempt is made to reduce the absolute level of sensory input to a minimum, which we call *deprivation;*
2) that in which the attempt is made to eliminate order and meaning from the sensory input, which we shall call *non-patterning.*

Heron adds a third category with regard to experimental conditions:

3) that in which the subject is exposed to some repeated stimulus figure against a patterned but fairly constant sensory background.

When our intent as clinicians who adhere to the auditory approach is to improve functional use of the auditory channel of hearing-impaired youngsters, perhaps one way of analyzing our task is to say that we are working within a sensitive period of development to overcome, to the greatest degree possible, effects of auditory deprivation, according to the definition of deprivation given above.

Heron considers central effects of sensory deprivation on the nervous system. Three types of effects are isolated primarily for academic purposes, for actually all of these effects are *inextricably interrelated:*

1) nonspecific effects, or those affecting the mechanisms concerned with the regulation of the electrical activity of the brain as a whole,
2) specific effects, which are more discrete and probably limited to a single sensory modality;
3) effects on whatever complex neural processes (phase sequences) underlie thought and action (Heron, 1961).

Two motivating factors concerning early identification and early therapeutic intervention of hearing loss can be derived from the above concepts. Obviously, one factor concerns the necessity for reversing effects of sensory deprivation. According to Bruner (1961):

Continued contact with a rich sensory environment . . . permits the development of differentiation of spheres of activity, of sensory modalities, of events within modalities. Sensory deprivation prevents such differentiation, prevents the development of selective gating.

The second motivating factor with regard to identification and intervention of hearing loss is directly related to time factors. We have been stressing the correlation of genetic and environmental interaction among developmental factors, supporting the notion of a sensitive period in which to effectively reach hearing-impaired children; however, there is reason to believe that a critical age factor, not merely a sensitive age factor, may exist with regard to reversing effects of auditory deprivation.

Since the mid-1950's, one of the most provocative findings of the HEAR Foundation has been that some hearing-impaired babies demonstrate remission of hearing loss at an average of five months following identification and therapy. The interim between detection of hearing impairment and remission has consisted of supplying auditory stimulation via binaural amplification and therapy specifically geared to teaching use of auditory input. Other components of the HEAR program include continuous exposure to normal speech and language models in a normal auditorally-saturated environment—sound sources which include, in addition to people, radios, televisions, phonographs, etc. Furthermore, one of the focuses of the program is working with parents to establish their involvement, cooperation and knowledge about the therapy employed.

In nearly twenty years, several thousand youngsters have been seen at the HEAR Foundation; of that number, 106 had entered the program prior to age eight months. Sixty-six of that 106, or 62 percent, have been able to discontinue use of hearing aids. The oldest child to demonstrate remission of hearing loss was eight months, three days of age upon entry into the Foundation.

In a recently completed three-year clinical investigation, 67 percent, 14 of 21, hearing-impaired infants who were younger than age eight months when therapy was initiated changed in a mean of 23.5 weeks (about five months) from indicating limited response to amplified sound to apparently normal hearing without amplification. None of the children whose therapy began between ages 8–24 months demonstrated audiometrically improved hearing levels. Functional use of hearing improved among children in the older group, which is felt to be consistent with the notion of sensitive period, but not one demonstrated remission of loss. (Ebbin and Griffiths, 1973)

Consistent with previous findings of the Foundation, none of the hearing loss remitters had been prenatal rubella infants. Among the remitters is a child whose mother is congenitally deaf and whose father was deafened by meningitis. Etiological reports from physicians had indicated that the child was probably congenitally deaf; yet within sixteen weeks following initiation of therapy, the child began to show normal responses to sound, both environmentally and audiometrically.

We have found no apparent relationship between specific age at initiation of therapy and remission time, as long as the child is within the first eight months of life.

We have found no apparent relationship between initial degree of hearing loss and remission time.

How is remission of hearing loss explained?

One obvious possibility is that the initial audiometric evaluation was in error. Several points would seem to mitigate against that notion:

1) There was a consistent lack of response on the part of all potential hearing loss remitters (and non-remitters) to both pure tone stimuli as well as complex environmental sounds.

2) Diagnosis of hearing-loss was confirmed by one or more physicians and occasionally by another hearing center prior to each child's entry into the program.

3) Hearing levels did not improve immediately upon the child's receipt of hearing aids; gradual changes in the functioning of the auditory channel could be observed during the course of therapy. In some instances, improvement was initially noted monaurally followed soon by the second ear's improved response to sound.

4) A control group for audiometric purposes only had been incorporated into the experimental design. The function of this group of normally hearing infants was to provide indication of the Foundation's diagnostic ability in identifying normal versus abnormal responses to sound. Initial diagnosis of normal hearing in each member of the control group was substantiated on subsequent and repeated evaluation. Thus, it was felt that the diagnosis of deafness among the experimental group subjects was probably accurate as well.

Assuming that initial audiometric evaluations were correct and that children in the experimental groups were indeed hearing-impaired, explanations of hearing loss remission, while still not definitive, fall somewhat less within the realm of an "impossible dream" than was so a decade ago. Is it likely that spontaneous remission might have occurred in all instances? The neurophysiological literature furnishes evidence in support of hearing loss remission possibilities.

Carter, an otologist offered the following theory:

> There may be some children who are born with an immature hearing mechanism which is not adequate to receive sound with sufficient competence, and therefore the central cortex is not stimulated . . . Stimulation by means of amplified sound results in the complete functional development of those neural pathways, and thus normal hearing develops. (Cited by Griffiths, 1967.)

Krmpotic, an anatomist, suggested that "complete myelination of the neural pathways of hearing is not possible for some infants because of a maturation lag, unless amplified sound is supplied soon after birth." Perhaps myelination becomes static by the eight month of life and accounts for the inability of infants older than this age to demonstrate hearing loss remission. (Cited by Griffiths, 1967.)

Galambos suggested that babies with remission of hearing loss probably had *intact wiring,* but for some physiological reason, had not been *turned on* to sound until auditory stimulation had been introduced. Work by Magoun (1954, 1963) and Lindsley (1961), among others, on the reticular activating system would seem to speak directly to Galambos' notion:

> This central reticular mechanism has been found capable of grading the activity of most other parts of the brain. It does this as a reflection of its own internal excitability, in turn a consequence of both afferent and corticifugal neural influences, as well as of the titer of circulating transmitters and hormones which affect and modify reticular activity.
>
> While the functions of this reticular system tend generally to be more widespread than those of the specific systems of the brain, it is proposed to be subdivided into a grosser and more tonically operating component in the lower brain stem, subserving global alterations in excitability . . . (Magoun, 1963).

The reticulo-cortical and cortico-reticular influences of this brain stem mechanism are intimately connected to initiation and maintenance of wakefulness, to the orienting reflex and attentional focuses, to sensory control processes which relate to selective gating, mentioned above in Bruner's discussion of effects of sensory deprivation, to conditional learning, to memory functions and to internal inhibition. "These manifold and varied capacities of the reticular system suggest that it serves importantly and in the closest conjunction with the cortex in most of the central integrative processes of the brain" (Magoun, 1963).

Consider the steps in auditory stimulation therapy for hearing impairment: first we teach awareness of sound, followed by auditory localization; thus, it appears logical to assume that in order to achieve auditory localization, the reticular activating system must be functionng. When we observe hearing loss remission, has the underlying problem been as a result of now-corrected brain stem malfunctioning?

Let us examine auditory localization from the vantage point of recent findings. Research in sensory physiology is cited which would appear to pinpoint the inferior colliculus and superior olivary complex as chief centers for the spatial analysis of sound. These centers are probably significant, as well, in simple frequency discrimination. Some medial geniculate neurons which are binaurally responsive may be important in fusion interval discrimination, laterality discrimination and in organizing input to the auditory cortex which indicates sound direction (Altman, 1971; Tamar, 1972). Are neurophysiological and neurochemical disturbances in these areas correctible?

Bjorklund and Stenevi, Swedish researchers, (1972) have reported their work with nerve-growth-factor effects on stimulating growth of central noradrenergic neurons: "Nerve growth factor (NGF) is a potent stimulator of growth of peripheral, sympathetic and sensory neurons . . . it is most effective on developing or growing neurons." This research is probably the first to demonstrate effects of NGF on central neurons. One of the suggestions is that NGF may be an 'endogenous, normally occurring physiological factor that is required for the normal development, maturation and growth of certain central neuron systems. . . ."

Lynch and Cotman (1973) report a highly pertinent study "demonstrating that the brain is capable of *rewiring* itself after injury." The particularly salient points of Lynch and Cotman's work with regard to hearing loss remission are that growth of nervous tissue left intact after brain damage is a process which occurs simultaneously in different brain systems, that it occurs in radically different ways depending upon the age of the animal and that measurements of the magnitude of the effect are possible (1973).

Teuber (1973), in a recent National Academy of Sciences address, cited results of research investigations which "suggest" that not all brain cells are already specialized at the time of birth, but may remain open to *instruction* for an undetermined period in early childhood. The challenge is to determine how long the period of brain plasticity lasts and at what point it *peaks*."

The compilation of all of the above points may, indeed, help to explain the possibility of hearing loss remission. What about the apparent critical age factor of eight months? Why is it that no child seen at the HEAR Foundation after the age of eight months has ever demonstrated hearing loss remission? Herein lies a particularly intriguing area of potential research. One animal study of auditory deprivation has been reported by Graven (1968). An eight-day critical age factor was found in a study of baby chicks. Comparison of the eight days versus eight months time periods to total life expectancy of each species reveals practically identical percentages, perhaps indicative of similar phenomena.

In summary, there appears to be a critical age factor associated with reversing a type of hearing impairment. Beyond a critical period, which seems to end at about age eight months in humans, for some babies who have been deprived of *adequate* sound, the possibility of reversing this hearing disorder may be eliminated. We in no way believe that a cure has been found for restoring function to damaged cochlear hair cells. Rather, it would appear more appropriate to hypothesize that another type of hearing deficit has been isolated. Further, it may be that once a critical period has been exceeded, retrospectively discriminating between potentially remissable and non-remissable hearing loss becomes impossible.

The scientific era in which we mutually participate is especially conducive to vigorous inquiry into mechanisms underlying a potentially critical age in hearing. *The definitive study proving hearing loss remission has yet to be done.* A research area in which we are presently involved concerns longitudinal studies of our hearing loss remitters and non-remitters to note incidence and type of auditory processing deficits among other signs of minimal brain dysfunction.

I shall conclude with an incentive to all of us who, in various contexts, determine the learning experiences of hearing-impaired children. Ragan and Shepherd's book, *Modern Elementary Curriculum*, (1971) cites work by David Krech, who has reported "recent findings of research in brain biochemistry and behavior which he believes may have favorable consequences for education. He says, 'Educators probably change brain structure and chemistry to a greater degree than any biochemist in the business.'" We need very much to know how and which brain mechanisms change in response to auditory stimulation.

BIBLIOGRAPHY

Altman, J.: Neurophysiological Mechanism of Soundsource Localization. In Gersuni, G. (Ed.): *Sensory Processes at the Neuronal and Behavioral Levels.* New York: Academic Press, 1971.

Bjorklund, A. and Stenevi, U.: Nerve growth factor: Stimulation of regenerative growth of central noradrenergic neurons. *Science, 175:*1251–1253, 1972.

Bruner, J.: The Cognitive Consequences of Early Sensory Deprivation. In Solomon, P. *et al.* (Eds.): *Sensory Deprivation.* Cambridge: Harvard University Press, 1961.

Ebbin, J. and Griffiths, S.: Effectiveness of Early Detection and Auditory Stimulation on the Speech and Language of Hearing-impaired Children. Contract No. HSM–110–69–413, Health Services and Mental Health Administration, Department of Health, Education and Welfare. To be published in 1973.

Freedman, S., Grunebaum, H. and Greenblatt, M.: Perceptual and Cognitive Changes in Sensory Deprivation. In Solomon, P. *et al.* (Eds.): *Sensory Deprivation.* Cambridge: Harvard University Press, 1961.

Galambos, R.: Personal communication. July 10, 1972. Robert Galambos, M.D., Ph.D., University of California School of Medicine, San Diego, California.

Graven, J.: *Non-human Thought.* London: Arlington Books, 1968.

Griffiths, C.: *Conquering Childhood Deafness.* New York: Exposition Press, 1967.

Heron, W.: Cognitive and Physiological Effects of Perceptual Isolation. In Solomon, P. *et al.* (Eds.): *Sensory Deprivation.* Cambridge: Harvard University Press, 1961.

Lewis, M.: *Clinical Aspects of Child Development.* Philadelphia: Lea and Febiger, 1971.

Lindsley, D.: Common Factors in Sensory Deprivation, Sensory Distortion and Sensory Overload. In Solomon, P. *et al.* (Eds.): *Sensory Deprivation.* Cambridge: Harvard University Press, 1961.

Lynch, G. and Cotman, C.: *University Bulletin* (University of California), *21:*92, January 1973.

Magoun, H.: The Ascending Reticular System and Wakefulness. In Delafresnaye, J. (Ed.): *Brain Mechanisms and Consciousness*. Oxford: Blackwell, 1954.

Magoun, H.: *The Waking Brain*. Springfield: Thomas, 1963.

Ragan, W. and Shepherd, G.: *Modern Elementary Curriculum*. New York: Holt, Rinehart and Winston, 1971.

Tamar, H.: *Principles of Sensory Physiology*. Springfield: Thomas, 1972.

Teuber, H.: *Today's Child*, 21:5, February 1973.

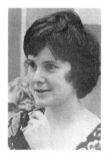

JUDITH EBBIN, M.A., M.S.

Judith Ebbin, Assistant Research Director of the HEAR Foundation, received her undergraduate education at Syracuse University. She holds a Master's Degree in Audiology and Speech Pathology from Syracuse and a Master's Degree in Developmental Psychology from the University of California, Los Angeles. She is completing doctoral studies at the University of Southern California. Her training as a teacher of the deaf was at the Clarke School for the Deaf. She has been associated with numerous programs for the deaf, deaf-blind, cerebral palsied and aphasic in Connecticut, Massachusetts, New York and California. She has presented papers at several professional meetings and has conducted seminars in the area of early-detection/early intervention of hearing loss. Among her areas of major professional interest are critical periods in development and language acquisition. Membership in professional organizations includes the American Speech and Hearing Association, Council for Exceptional Children, California Association for Neurologically Handicapped Children and the California Speech and Hearing Association. Mrs. Ebbin holds the Certificate of Clinical Competence in Audiology and in Speech Pathology, granted by the American Speech and Hearing Association.

Chapter X

AUDITORY TECHNIQUES IN A LARGE SCHOOL POPULATION

TYLER HAYES

THE ABOVE TITLE is great, but let me the first to admit that all of the auditory techniques that we know about and are now available are not in use. We do not have enough money. We do not have enough trained personnel. And, in the area of the deaf and hard of hearing, we are faced with the same dilemmas that have been in existence for years.

However, it can honestly be reported that the *Los Angeles Unified City School District* is working on the problems that do exist and, in spite of our size, a year from now will be able to report that more and better educational programs are being provided for our deaf and hard of hearing pupils.

Perhaps we are fortunate! There is no school system in the nation that is more subject to change than Los Angeles City. Not only do we have a federal government that is presently creating change, but we also have a state legislature that is constantly requiring change. In addition to the change required by the federal and state governments, there are those of us working within the District that still think that by trying some new ideas, we can hopefully provide better programs which come closer to meeting the needs of all our pupils whether they be handicapped or not.

Let me reiterate. To quote what some of you have put on tape, or perhaps what some of you may read at a later date, it would be a mistake to quote whatever I might say, for what is being stated today will not be the case tomorrow.

This matter of change is important enough to discuss even further. At the present time, all programs in Special Education, including the deaf and hard of hearing, are presently in a rapid state of transition in California.

Within the past year, a State Level Master Plan has been formulated for all of special education. Fortunately, this new Master Plan is based upon the continued moral commitments, legislative mandate and public

81

policy of this state. It is a mandate that *all pupils be provided an education appropriate to their needs.*

Perhaps there are those that would equate *bigness with badness.* If this were truly the case, many of us who are still deeply concerned with individual pupil needs would have handed in our resignations a long time ago. Many times the frustrations are great. However, with strong and supportive help from the administration, there are new, innovative and educationally sound programs being introduced all the time. (After all, if *big were bad,* why are there so many of us driving General Motors automobiles?)

In discussing techniques, one must first discuss philosophy. Because of our bigness, we should be able to offer a more diversified program to meet individual needs. (And possibly no disability exerts an impact on so many aspects of a child's development as does a hearing impairment.) Intelligence, language, oral communication, school achievement, general adjustment and ability to relate all tend to be adversely affected. But these are no real measure of a child's potential or human worth; therefore, it is to the advantage of society and the child that he be provided with the most skilled instruction possible.

Technique must involve suitable placement, and this is done based upon (1) the amount of hearing loss, (2) onset, etiology and stability of loss, (3) communication skills, (4) past educational experiences and, out of necessity, (5) a consideration for the location of residence—at least in a district as far-flung as the Los Angeles City School System.

Technique has to involve what the classroom teacher has available to use. *Electronic auditory training equipment is given top priority.* This is followed by a multi-media approach to teaching the latest curriculum concepts to individualize each pupil's instruction. Mrs. Lois Tarkanian, Director of *Oralingua School for the Deaf,* talked so succinctly of the need for "Integration: Purpose and Practice." *The deaf and hard of hearing pupils must be made a part of the mainstream wherever and whenever possible!*

Perhaps the most important technique is to offer proper placement for a child—*placement where he can succeed!* Such placement must be constantly evaluated in terms of progress. If there is a need for further diagnosis and/or re-assessment, it should be done! (And this should be done not according to what the law requires, but according to the child's needs!) I sincerely feel that our District is doing a better job of this all the time.

As part of my own job responsibilities, I serve as a member of what is called a Placement Committee. The Committee tries to make the best possible placement for each pupil. Placement information is: (1) a child's physical and medical history, including any and all information regarding his hearing; (2) a complete psychological work-up along with pertinent in-put concerning the child's environmental background and (3) when required for placement, a complete work-up done by a speech, language and hearing specialist concerning the level of the child's speech and language development in the areas of phonology, morphology, syntax and semantics. Because of our school population, test scores on standardized tests are not weighed as heavily as other information presented at the Placement Committee meetings. (I am specifically speaking of those pupils who come from a bilingual and/or bidialectical background.) Placement of every pupil is only made after careful consideration of all information. It is the decision of the whole committee and *not* the decision of one member.

Rules and regulations have too often dictated where a child is to be placed. If it is a technique, proper placement is perhaps the most difficult. All school systems have made mistakes for there is no perfect formula. The younger the child, the more difficult it is to make placement. There is no panacea, but many of us presently feel that there should be a *diagnostic class* where the medical, psychological and language assessments are an on-going process in terms of deciding the best possible educational placement for a child. For some children, decisions may be reached in a matter of a few weeks. For others, even after careful logging of all aspects of a child's behavior, there still may be real question marks as to where we can place the child to best meet his educational needs. Let me repeat—there is no panacea!

Since we are now aware of the fact that proper placement is preceded only by most careful diagnosis and assessment, let us take a look at what the available programs for the hearing-impaired child in a large school population are.

In Los Angeles City Schools, there are presently 156 speech, language and hearing specialists working in over 550 schools in the District. Sixty-six of these specialists work on a regular schedule, using auditory trainers for pupils who are functioning with mild to moderate hearing losses in regular school settings. These specialists are offering an auxiliary service in language development, speech reading, tutorial assistance and/or articulation therapy. These are services provided by the speech and hearing department. This department serves both needs of the regular elementary and secondary divisions of the District but, in addition, also serves the needs of all the schools in the Special Education Division.

However, this is only a beginning concerning the present programs and services now being offered. Not only is the Special Education Division the largest in any school system in the nation, but also the Deaf and Hard of Hearing Program is the largest in the United States. Los Angeles City

School District covers 711 square miles, and in the Deaf and Hard of Hearing Program at the present time, over 900 hearing-impaired children are being served.

We know there are more pupils that we have either not been made aware of, and/or they have not been assessed properly in terms of their needs. This is our most important consideration at the present time—to find those we have missed and to change those that have been placed inappropriately and/or need a change of placement. This in and of itself is a major task in a district the size of Los Angeles City.

Technique, however, is to recognize needs and offer a wide variety of programs. We have already discussed those pupils that are served by the speech, language and hearing specialists. But the District is now offering several other most worthwhile programs for the hearing-impaired pupils—programs which have already proved their worth and desparately need expansion based upon their success.

THE ITINERANT TEACHER PROGRAM. This program is presently serving 56 pupils with mild to profound losses. These pupils are in their own local school, and they are able to compete academically as well as socially. The itinerant teacher provides enough assistance to make this possible for those children who do not need full time special classes or special school placement. The itinerant teacher sees each child two or three times a week individually and works with the regular school staff. In some cases, even the speech, language and hearing specialist serving the school will work in close coordination with the itinerant teacher and the staff. The needs of the child are the determining factors when it comes to creating the best possible program for the hearing-impaired child.

How can anyone help but agree with Dr. Ciwa Griffiths when she says that these children should be kept in a regular school setting, functioning as normally as possible in a hearing world. They need maximum amplification, and it should be our primary concern to see that they have it and on a regular basis. This means that their own personal equipment should be checked whenever there is any indication to do so, either by the pupil or by the way he does or does not respond; it has nothing to do with the laws and regulations as to how often he should be checked and by whom, etc.

THE INTEGRATED PROGRAM. The Los Angeles City School District also offers an Integrated Program, which provides classes for deaf and hard of hearing children in regular elementary and secondary schools. Pupils are served by a special teacher of the deaf but attend selected classes with hearing pupils depending upon individual needs and abilities. They also participate in school activities with hearing students.

There are also three special schools for hearing-impaired children. These special schools provide full time classes for hearing-impaired children. All of these schools offer complete programs for children from preschool through age twenty-one.

In addition, there is also a program for the deaf-blind.

If the programs offered are to function effectively, then it is most important that constant reevaluation take place so that every pupil be given the opportunity to move from one program to another based upon his need.

It is now also possible to discuss audiological services within the district. *The Special Education Division* now has the services of an educational audiologist. Services provided by the educational audiologist include: (1) audiological evaluations and interpretations to teachers, parents and administrators, (2) evaluation of student-classroom amplification equipment and recommendations for district purchases and maintenance agreements and (3) instruction to classroom teachers on the effective use of the auditory avenue in teaching the hearing-impaired.

In addition to all of the above mentioned programs, there are curriculum teachers who serve the special schools and the integrated classes. Their responsibility is to introduce new material and techniques to the classroom and serve as liaison between special teachers.

There are also vocational education programs which provide instructional programs in community training facilities and work with the *California Department of Vocational Rehabilitation*.

We are a large public school system, serving a very large school population. We are not the best, but we are working toward it. If everyone in attendance at this Conference would come to us with their knowledge and their constructive criticism, perhaps some day in the not too distant future, I can say in my opening remarks that "all of the auditory techniques that we know about and are now available, are being used to serve our large school population."

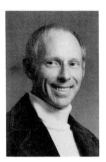

TYLER S. HAYES, M.A.

Mr. Tyler S. Hayes is Speech and Hearing Specialist, Special Education Division, Los Angeles City School District. Mr. Hayes received his B.A. Degree from Allegheny College in Meadville, Pennsylvania in 1955 and his Masters from C.S.U.L.A. in Los Angeles, California in 1965. He has served as a secondary teacher of English and reading for two years and has been an Elementary and Secondary Speech/Hearing Therapist Los Angeles City School Districts for the past nine years, becoming an administrative specialist of the Speech and Hearing Program for the Los Angeles City School District (East and South Areas) for the past four years.

In addition to the work with Los Angeles City School District, Mr. Hayes has additional experience as consultant and teacher of Speech and Language Development for the Trainable Mentally Retarded Program, Assistant Professor at C.S.U.L.A. in the Audiology Clinic and a guest lecturer Speech/Hearing Program, University of New Mexico. He holds a certificate for Clinical Competency, American Speech and Hearing Association and is past president for the Council of Exceptional Children.

Mr. Hayes is vice president, program chairman and membership chairman for the California Speech/Hearing Association and is presently associate editor for the "State Journal." He has authored two articles: "California State Journal of Communicative Disorders" and served as Special Education Consultant to Columbia Broadcasting Company Educational Films Division and a chairman for Special Education Legislation Committee, Los Angeles City.

Chapter XI

AUDITORY TECHNIQUES IN ISRAEL

ETHEL COHEN

THE NON-SELECTIVITY of the MICHA[1] program for preschool deaf and severely hard of hearing children lends itself well to analyzing the factors which are the most crucial in the development of oral communication. Every child referred to us is accepted in our program almost immediately, regardless of socio-economic family background, initial ability of the parents to actively participate in the program, visible or probable additional problems. Our belief is that all deaf babies will benefit from our program with varying degrees of success and that all parents of deaf children need constant guidance and encouragement, for in the final analysis they are the children's teachers. Those families who cannot actively participate, such as deaf parents, parents of very large families where time and energy must be sustained for many children and recent immigrant families, must be provided with some help at home so that their deaf children, too, will have the carry-over in the home from the center.

Most of our children are referred to us between the ages of twelve and eighteen months. This is in stark contrast to the time, only a few years ago, when most children were referred between two and three years of age. The babies who are referred to us between the ages of five and twelve months are predominantly the high-risk babies whose parents are deaf, who have deaf siblings, the premature and rubella baby. Mass screening of hearing of new born infants, which is being done in a few hospitals, has led to earlier referral of infants to the MICHA program, after the suspect cases have been periodically retested.

The babies who are accepted into the program are fitted with their own binaural hearing aids, generally within three months after admission. In the interim, they are fittted with aids loaned to them by the center. Audiology centers are still rather cautious about recommending hearing aids to babies under the age of ten to twelve months and feel more con-

---

[1] The name *MICHA* is derived from the initials of the Hebrew words meaning *educators of deaf children*. MICHA is a voluntary agency organized in 1956 by a group of parents and an otologist, Dr. Ezra Korine. The first director-teacher was Dr. Jerome Reichstein.

fident only after the baby has been in the MICHA program for a few months, has had auditory training with the use of amplification and is then retested with his own teacher assisting.

The baby and his mother (father, too, whenever possible) come to the center twice a week for individual tutoring until the age of two. During the past few years, we have taught some of the babies in their own homes during the first year of training. In the opinion of this writer, the advantages of having the parents come to the center for the child's training is greater. We do recommend, however, that during this first year, periodic visits to the home by the child's teacher or other staff member to check on situational suggestions which have been made to parents, to observe the baby at home and to offer on the spot guidance to the parents. Some of our babies, upon the recommendation of our social worker who visits every home at least once during the first year, attend a normal nursery or day care center close to their home from the age of twelve months. This is especially desirable for babies of deaf parents, culturally deprived and new immigrant families, who cannot give their babies the auditory stimulation and language learning they require.

From the age of two to four, the children attend the MICHA center nursery school twice a week and continue to receive individual therapy during the morning hours. The parents continue to observe the individual lessons and the child in the nursery set up through observation mirrors. Every week one mother works in the nursery under the supervision of the nursery school teacher. There are generally eight children in each group. During the other four days, these children continue to attend a normal nursery or kindergarten. Attendance at a day care center, nursery school and kindergarten is the first step in the carefully structured integrated program which is carefully planned and supervised for each child.

The nursery and kindergarten staff receive specific guidance and training from one of the MICHA teachers who visits the kindergarten for this purpose. An orientation program is conducted in the MICHA center every year for all the personnel who have deaf children in their groups. The orientation program consists of at least ten hours of lectures, demonstration lessons and discussion periods and has proven invaluable in enlisting their support and interest. Some of these teachers, as a result of this contact and experience, have since entered the field of special education of the deaf.

Between the ages of four and seven, the children are in a government-supported, integrated kindergarten consisting of 24 hearing children with a group of eight deaf children. This program is conducted by two trained kindergarten teachers and the MICHA tutor who continues to give individual therapy to each child. The emphasis in the program is intensive, individual work in auditory training, speech and language development, conceptual learning, reading and social integration. We have experimented with different ratios of deaf and hearing children with little discernable differences in the children's progress. The ratio of three to four hearing children to one deaf child with no more than six to eight deaf children in any one group seems to be a good proportion. Of course, the smaller the number of children in the total group, the more opportunities for more individualized programming. For many children, this intensive, daily, integrated program has often yielded results far above our expectations.

Certainly, the factors most responsible for successful oral communication seem to be the ability of the child to utilize his residual hearing with amplification, the ability to develop lipreading skill, his intelligence and motivation. Basically important is the early age at which the child is exposed to amplification and the auditory learning program. Also basically important is the consistent supportive help of the parents. To ensure this support from the very start and all during the four to six years that the child is in our program, the parents are in a structured guidance program.

In addition to observing their child's individual lessons and the nursery program, the parents are expected to attend the introductory course for parents in the evenings during the first two years. This is an 18- to 20-hour course consisting of lectures by staff teachers, psychologists, psychiatrists and guest lecturers such as otologists, audiologists and pediatricians. At many of these meetings, *graduate* parents participate in panels. This is of tremendous importance for in addition to getting the scientific cold facts from the specialists, they have the opportunity to hear from other parents how they, themselves, worked with their children, "that it can succeed." The encouragement and know-how they get from such meetings is invaluable. The staff social worker visits the home of every child to learn first hand the home situation, to assess the amount of support the parents will need and to offer guidance. This year, our consultant psychiatrist is conducting a series of parent guidance sessions with small groups of no more than eight to ten parents in the morning hours, as well as seeing individual parents for which special guidance help is recommended. The entire auditory learning program, the consistent correct use of the hearing aids, is all dependent on parent acceptance and support. It is important and often difficult to find and maintain the delicate balance between getting maximum parental cooperation and avoiding excess pressure which some parents are prone to exert on their children.

Upon completion of the preschool program, most of the children are placed in integrated elementary school programs. The largest number go into small classes of six to eight children in a normal school and integrate with the parallel hearing class in certain subjects such as art and gymnastics. Eventually some of the children may spend one hour or more in the parallel hearing class. Each child will integrate according to his own ability. A few children are placed in hearing classes where the ratio may be 25 hearing to three or four deaf children. Still a few others are placed in a full-capacity hearing class. There are the children who have made superior progress in oral communication, have good social orientation and whose parents are able to provide them with additional help both in schoolwork and speech therapy. Every deaf child who is in a hearing class is provided with three hours per week additional help by law. The children who are multiple-handicapped, whose parents could not provide any home support and for whom volunteer supplementary help was not enough are placed in the school for the deaf.

The importance of providing an orientation program for the teachers and other staff members of the integrated schools is self evident but has still not been done. The MICHA staff has recognized this need and invites many of these teachers both to parent meetings and the orientation program for kindergarten teachers, but this is not enough for them.

I do not believe that the simultaneous method or total communication approach, as it is now known, of teaching the deaf is valid at the preschool level. I do believe that if we have faith in the auditory approach, are able to start to work with the child at a very early age, keep the child in a hearing environment all during the preschool years and give the parents the much needed guidance and training, our total results would be consistently better. How can the auditory approach be criticized by educators who did not insist on early amplification, did not keep the children in a hearing environment and did not program intensive parent guidance to ensure home reinforcement? There are some educators and psychologists who imply that the auditory learning approach and oralism is for hard-of-hearing children. If we prejudged the ability of our children to learn to communicate orally on the basis of their auditory thresholds, we would be denying many, perhaps most, deaf children the chance to learn to communicate orally. The fact is that many of our children with severe hearing losses are communicating orally, with pleasant and understandable speech.

I am certain that we have not yet explored every avenue which will help the deaf child to achieve better oral communication, to reach his intellectual potential and to integrate more fully into the hearing society. We must be constantly on the alert to new ideas, be flexible enough to apply new methods and new equipment and to take the time to periodically study and evaluate the progress of every child with the purpose of seeking and applying reinforcement wherever it is needed.

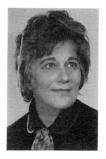

ETHEL COHEN, B.S., M.A.

Mrs. Cohen was born in the United States and received her Bachelor of Science Degree in psychology and speech at Hunter College in New York in 1936. She worked with the Lexington School for the Deaf in their teacher-training program in education for the deaf from 1957 through 1959. She received her Masters in special education (Education of the Deaf) Columbia University, New York, in 1959. Mrs. Cohen was assistant director at the MICHA Preschool Center for Deaf Children and Parents and teacher at that school from 1959 to 1965 and in 1965 was appointed director of the MICHA Center. She has been instrumental in setting up the centers for preschool training and guidance programs in Ashdod, Haifa, Beersheba and Jerusalem.

Mrs. Cohen is a member of the faculty at Tel-Aviv University School of Communication Disorders. She is supervising teacher and has presented papers on preschool education of the deaf at the International Congress for Educators of the Deaf in 1963 in Washington, D.C. and in Stockholm, Sweden in 1970.

Mrs. Cohen is married and has 2 children and has been residing in Israel since 1951.

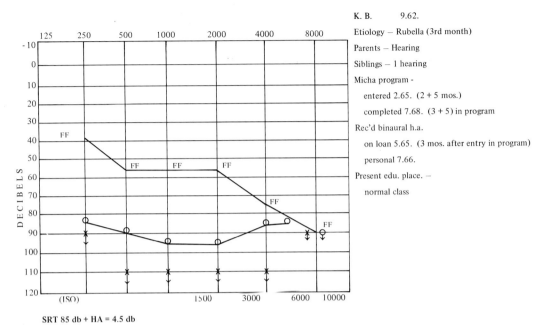

K. B.   9.62.

Etiology – Rubella (3rd month)

Parents – Hearing

Siblings – 1 hearing

Micha program -

    entered 2.65. (2 + 5 mos.)

    completed 7.68. (3 + 5) in program

Rec'd binaural h.a.

    on loan 5.65. (3 mos. after entry in program)

    personal 7.66.

Present edu. place. –

    normal class

SRT 85 db + HA = 4.5 db

Figure XI-1

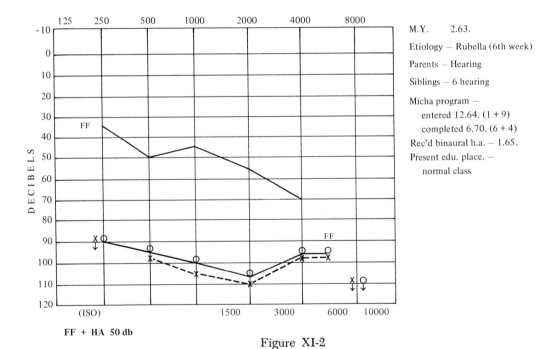

M.Y.   2.63.

Etiology – Rubella (6th week)

Parents – Hearing

Siblings – 6 hearing

Micha program –

    entered 12.64. (1 + 9)

    completed 6.70. (6 + 4)

Rec'd binaural h.a. – 1.65.

Present edu. place. –

    normal class

FF + HA 50 db

Figure XI-2

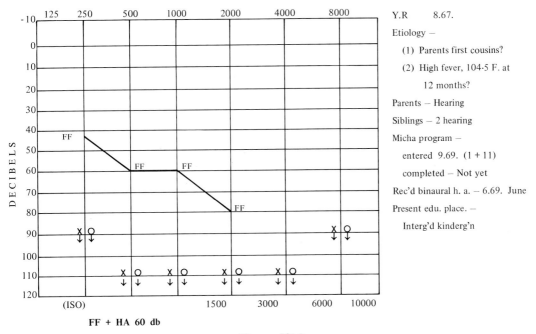

FF + HA 60 db

Figure XI-3

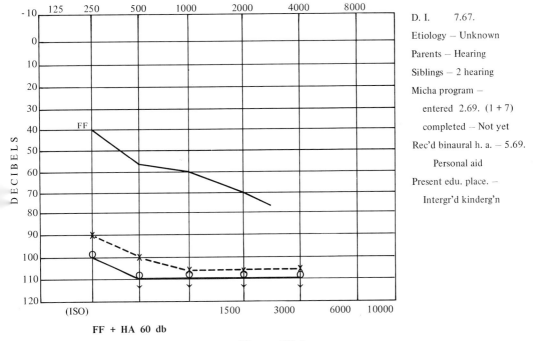

FF + HA 60 db

Figure XI-4

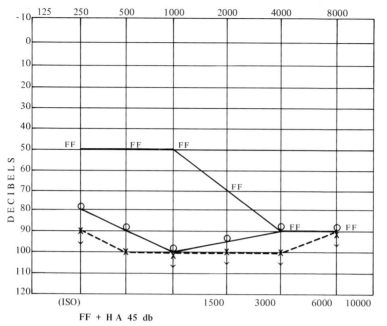

FF + H A 45 db

Right: 250 - 90   500 - 95   1000 - 105   2000 - 100   4000 - 100   8000 - 85
Left: 250 - 90   500 - 100 1000 - 105   2000 - 110   4000 - 105   8000 - 85

Figure XI-5

D.M.   8.62.
Etiology – Rubella (4th month)
Parents – Hearing
Siblings – 3 hearing
Micha program –
    entered 9.64. (2 + 1)
    completed 6.69. (6 + 10)
Rec'd binaural h.a. – 7.64.
Present edu. place. –
    normal class

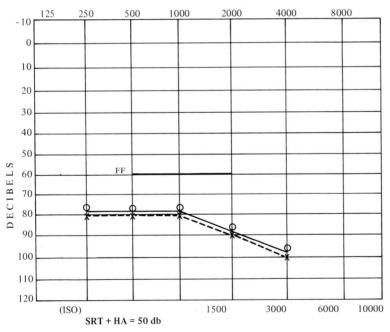

SRT + HA = 50 db

Right: 250 -   500 - 105   1000 - 90   2000 - 95   4000 - 90
Left: 250 -   500 - 105   1000 - 100   2000 - 90   4000 - 85

Figure XI-6

L. S.   1.63. (10 years)
Etiology – Rubella, also
    has severe vision loss
Parents – Hearing
Siblings – 1 hearing
Micha program –
    entered 5.64., left,
        reentered 9.66.
    completed Not yet 1969
Rec'd binaural h.a. – 1.67.
Present edu. place. –
    normal class 4th grade

Vision Loss

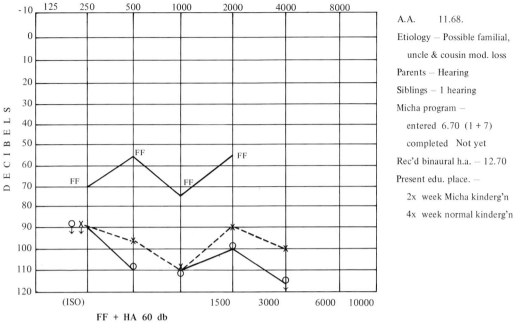

FF + HA 60 db

A.A.   11.68.

Etiology — Possible familial,
   uncle & cousin mod. loss

Parents — Hearing

Siblings — 1 hearing

Micha program —
   entered 6.70 (1 + 7)
   completed   Not yet

Rec'd binaural h.a. — 12.70

Present edu. place. —
   2x week Micha kinderg'n
   4x week normal kinderg'n

Figure XI-7

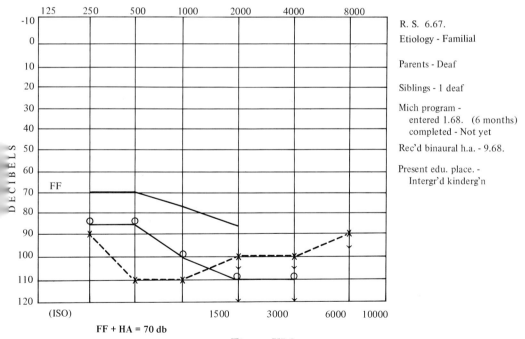

FF + HA = 70 db

R. S. 6.67.

Etiology - Familial

Parents - Deaf

Siblings - 1 deaf

Mich program -
   entered 1.68. (6 months)
   completed - Not yet

Rec'd binaural h.a. - 9.68.

Present edu. place. -
   Intergr'd kinderg'n

Figure XI-8

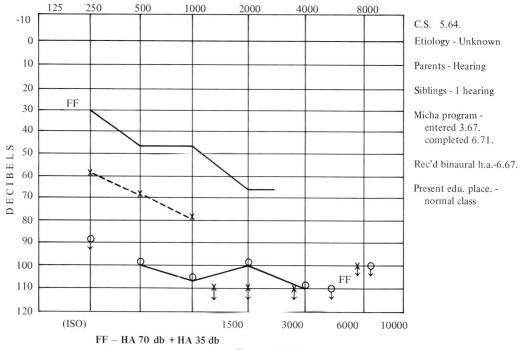

FF – HA 70 db + HA 35 db

Figure XI-9

C.S. 5.64.

Etiology - Unknown

Parents - Hearing

Siblings - 1 hearing

Micha program -
    entered 3.67.
    completed 6.71.

Rec'd binaural h.a.-6.67.

Present edu. place. -
    normal class

Chapter XII

SEQUENTIAL PROCESSING IN HEARING-IMPAIRED CHILDREN*

AGNES H. LING

ACCORDING TO Norman (1970), memory is viewed as a complex system of information processing involving three different types of storage system a sensory information store, a short-term memory and a long-term memory. Input from the environment is first registered by one or more of the sensory systems. For example, visual information is available very briefly in the form of an image (Sperling, 1960; 1963). Auditory information is available for a slightly longer duration at this precategorical acoustic level (Crowder and Morton, 1969). Neisser (1967) proposed the terms *iconic* and *echoic* for these sensory stores. Information at this level deteriorates rapidly unless categorized and entered into the short-term store where it comes under conscious control. The short-term store is also known as primary or working memory (Craik, 1971; Atkinson and Shiffrin, 1971) and is of very limited capacity. The basic processes operating in short-term memory appear to be rehearsal, coding, decision and retrieval strategies. Material can be retained in the short-term store only if it is rehearsed and organized in some way and if no other demands are made on the subject. Analysis of confusions indicates that many types of visual-verbal material are coded in auditory form (Conrad, 1964). New information entering the short-term store will replace old, and the latter will be forgotten if it has not been integrated into the long-term or permanent store. The long-term store represents our past experience, including our knowledge of language and thus can obviously affect the efficiency of rehearsal and coding strategies in short-term memory (Broadbent, 1971). The literature relating to auditory sequences has been competently reviewed by Aaronson (1967).

Visual Memory in Hearing-Impaired Children

As long ago as 1917, Pintner and Paterson found that deaf children had a very limited visual memory span for digits. A similar deficiency was

* The preparation of this paper was supported by Canadian Health Grant 604–7–725 to Dr. Daniel Ling. Research by the author quoted above was supported by Canadian Health Grant 604–7–72–729 to Dr. D.G. Doehring.

found more recently (Blair, 1957; Olsson and Furth, 1966). Poor recall of material presented visually has also been found to extend to other types of verbal material such as written sentences (Brill and Orman, 1953), sequences of words (Odom and Blanton, 1967) and sequences of letters (Conrad, 1970; Hartung, 1970). Whereas normal-hearing children were more efficient in recalling digit sequences in the given, rather than in the reverse order, hearing-impaired subjects showed equal recall on the two tasks (Blair, 1957). A similar finding for grammatical versus ungrammatical sequences of words was reported by Odom and Blanton (1967).

Findings relative to nonverbal sequences are conflicting. Blair (1957) found that hearing-impaired were superior to normal-hearing children on the recall of patterns of movement (Knox Cube Test) and on memory for designs. No significant differences between hearing-impaired and normal-hearing adolescent subjects were found for sequences of nonsense shapes (Olsson and Furth, 1966; Powell, 1971). A similar finding for children was obtained by Ross (1969) for sequentially presented series, nine items long, composed of two, three or four different symbols (plus, minus, square, circle). In contrast, Withrow (1968) found that when presentation of shapes was successive rather than simultaneous, when sequences were long and when presentation was rapid, hearing-impaired children were poorer than control subjects. Hearing-impaired subjects were also found to perform less well when recall was delayed rather than immediate (Goetzinger and Huber, 1964; DiFrancesca, 1969). Apparently hearing-impaired subjects can equal or surpass normal-hearing subjects in recalling certain types of visual sequences under certain conditions; for example, when a spatial coding strategy is effective and when neither group is experienced in the experimental task; however, normal-hearing children have an advantage in any recall task, either verbal or nonverbal, for which the most efficient strategy is one which involves verbal coding or rehearsal.

Auditory Perception of Temporal Order

In a classic series of studies, Hirsh (1959) found that whereas a delay in onset of about two msec. was sufficient for experienced subjects to detect that two sounds were present, a delay of approximately 20 msec. was required for their order to be perceived correctly 75 percent of the time. Hirsh used nonverbal stimuli such as pure tones and narrow-band noises. To detect the number of sounds in a longer sequence, however, greater temporal separation is required (White and Cheatham, 1959). Most of the research on temporal order has involved nonverbal stimuli; yet, on the basis of such data, generalizations have been made with respect to the perception of temporal order in speech. This weakness was pointed out by Fay (1966). He demonstrated that for phoneme pairs such as m/r, temporal order could be determined with an onset disparity of 10 msec., in comparison with at least 30 msec. required for the ordering of pure tone pairs by his inexperienced subjects.

The perception of the order of three or four unrelated sounds was studied by Warren and co-workers (Warren, Obusek, Farmer and Warren, 1969; Warren and Warren, 1970; Warren and Obusek, 1972). The sounds used in most of their experiments were a high tone (1000 Hz), a hiss (2000 Hz octave band noise), a low tone (796 Hz) and a buzz (40 Hz square wave). Each sound was followed by the next, without any inter-stimulus interval and played over and over without pause. When an oral response was required, an item duration of 670 msec. was needed for correct identification of temporal order. For a card-ordering response, 300 msec. was required.

A similar approach was used by Thomas, Hill, Carroll and Garcia (1970) to study the ability of listeners to perceive the order of vowel sounds. They used the vowels /i/e/a/u/ since these were distinctive both from a perceptual and an articulatory viewpoint and thus unlikely to be confused with one another. They found that with vowel segments of 125 msec. or more, subjects could obtain almost perfect scores. This contrasts with the results of Warren and his colleagues for nonverbal sounds.

Verbal and Nonverbal Auditory Perception

Experiments such as those reported above provide considerable support for the view that adult listeners have special facility for identifying the temporal order of speech as compared with nonspeech sequences. Indications of a verbal-nonverbal dichotomy are also to be found in the literature relating to cerebral laterality and the perception of speech and nonspeech sounds (Kimura, 1961a, b; 1964; 1967; Milner, 1962). Kimura applied the dichotic listening technique (Broadbent, 1954) in which pairs of competing stimuli are delivered to the two ears. Numerous investigations have supported Kimura's view that superior right-ear recall of digits, words and nonsense syllables may be accepted as indicating that speech mechanisms are lateralized in the left hemisphere, while the greater left-ear accuracy for the recall of melodic patterns and environmental sounds indicates the specialization of the right hemisphere in processing nonverbal sounds. Shankweiler and Studdert-Kennedy (1967) found that consonants in synthetic speech syllables were more strongly lateralized to the right ear than were vowels. Further experiments using natural consonant-vowel-consonant syllables (Studdert-Kennedy and Shankweiler, 1970) confirmed and extended these findings to include lateralization of the articulatory features of voicing and place of production in stop consonants in the dominant hemisphere. They proposed that:

> Specialization of the dominant hemisphere in speech perception is due to its possession of a linguistic coding device, not to specialized capacities for auditory analysis . . . while the general auditory system common to both hemispheres is equipped to extract the auditory parameters of a speech signal, the dominant hemisphere may be specialized for the extraction of linguistic features from those parameters (p. 579).

Auditory Sequencing Ability in Hearing-Impaired Children

Research on the perception of the temporal order of auditory events has generally been undertaken with adults. Some information about how normal hearing children process auditory sequences is available from studies which were principally concerned with persons having speech and language disorders (Aten and Davis, 1968; Ebbin and Edwards, 1967; Goodglass, Berko-Gleason and Hyde, 1970; Rosenthal, 1970; Winitz, 1969).

Furth and Pufall (1966) appear to have been the first workers to study the identification of auditory sequences by hearing-impaired children. They were principally concerned with the visual sequencing ability of children who were also aphasic. Normal-hearing, hearing-impaired and aphasic subjects aged six and ten years were studied. The auditory stimuli were (A) a white noise and (B) an organ tone from the middle octave. Both were easily discriminated by all but two young aphasic subjects. Six three-item sequences were constructed, each containing the two stimuli, e.g. BBA. The child's task was to associate each sequence with a number printed on a card. Differences between normal and hearing-impaired subjects in auditory sequencing were obscured by the grouping of data relating to hearing-impaired and aphasic children in the analysis of results.

The perception of nonverbal auditory sequences by hearing-impaired and normal-hearing children aged four to ten years was studied by Affolter (1970). Sequences were constructed from acoustic stimuli which varied in frequency (130 to 500 Hz), intensity (20 or 30 dB SL) or both. Each element in an auditory sequence was one-half second and interstimulus intervals were of the same duration. Subjects indicated whether two given sequences were the same or different. At all age levels, and with all types of sequence, normal-hearing children were found to be superior.

The ability of 19 hearing-impaired children aged six to fourteen years to recall tape-recorded digit sequences was studied by A.H. Ling (1971) and found to be extremely poor in comparison with that of normal-hearing subjects, even among subjects with good auditory discrimination, indicating problems of processing sequences.

A subsequent experiment (A.H. Ling, 1972) was designed to investigate the ability of hearing-impaired and normal-hearing children to identify auditory sequences in relation to the type of stimulus (verbal or nonverbal), the rate of presentation and the length of sequence. It was predicted that certain of these factors would interact.

The verbal stimuli were two classes of speech sounds: syllables with different vowels /pi/pɛ/pa/po/pu/ and syllables with different consonants /la/ta/ma/ga/ʃa/. The nonverbal sounds were 200-msec. segments of environmental sounds, 200 msec. being the approximate duration of a syllable: a dog barking, a gun, a car horn, a sheep, and a mouse. Meaningful sounds were selected since, according to Gibson (1966), they are more distinctive and thus more readily perceived by the auditory system than pure tones or buzzes which are simple, artificial and meaningless. Tape-recorded sequences were constructed using each type of stimulus. Sequences of two, three and four items were prepared at each of the presentation rates, one, two and four items per second.

A nonverbal response was required for the nonverbal task, subjects being asked to point to the picture representing the sound they heard. For the verbal task, a verbal response was required. In this case, subjects had to repeat the syllables heard. A tape-recorded screening test of single items was used to select subjects who were able to repeat the syllables distinctly and point to the pictures representing the nonverbal sounds. Eighteen hearing-impaired subjects with residual hearing across the range of speech frequencies met the criteria. They were aged 6–14 years. Two groups of normal-hearing subjects were studied: 18 five-year-olds and 18 nine-year-olds.

Verbal sequences were more accurately identified than nonverbal sequences by normal-hearing subjects aged five and nine years, the vowel sequences being easier than the consonant sequences for the younger group. For the 18 hearing-impaired subjects, the vowel sequences were easier than the nonverbal sequences, while consonant sequences were poorly recalled.

Both groups of normal-hearing children were superior to the hearing-impaired group on both verbal tasks, but on the nonverbal task only the older group was superior to the hearing-impaired group. The latter were significantly better at recalling nonverbal sequences than were normal-hearing five-year-olds.

For hearing-impaired subjects, the longer the sequence, the less well it was recalled, whereas for normal-hearing subjects an increase in length had little effect on the recall of verbal sequences but caused a marked reduction in the recall of nonverbal sequences.

The optimal rate of presentation was found to vary according to the

type of material to be recalled. The fast, four-item per second rate fa-
cilitated consonant recall, while the slow, one-item per second rate proved
to be most appropriate for nonverbal sequences. Vowel sequences were
well recalled at all three rates. These results were consistent for hearing-
impaired as well as for normal-hearing children. Presentation rate has
previously been found to affect the accuracy and the strategies adopted
by adult listeners in auditory recall tasks (Aaronson, 1968; Cole, Sales
and Haber, 1969). For verbal sequences, the children had the advantage
of being highly practiced. Although the hearing-impaired children were
able to perceive and identify the syllables when they occurred singly,
their recall of sequences was poor. This may have been because they
were unable to perceive and identify new items while retaining earlier
items. Only a limited time is available in a short-term memory task and
has to be shared among several processes (Aaronson, 1967; Shulman, 1971;
Massaro, 1970). Weakness of auditory/articulatory coding probably prevents the development of automatic auditory-vocal sequencing noted
among normal-hearing children.

Neither normal-hearing nor hearing-impaired subjects had had any
previous experience and therefore had no ready-made strategies for processing sequences of environmental sounds. Three different strategies were
observed: covert naming, mimicking of sounds and the use of spatial
cues. The latter appeared to be used very effectively by some hearing-
impaired subjects. Covert naming was used by both normal-hearing and
hearing-impaired subjects but was appropriate only for the slower rate.
The preference for spatial, rather than temporal, organization of events
by hearing-impaired children has also been reported by O'Connor and
Hermelin (1972).

The results for nonverbal sequences support the view (Furth and
Youniss, 1969; Ross, 1969) that hearing-impaired children can perform as
well as their normal-hearing counterparts when the task is equally unfamiliar to both groups and when auditory or linguistic coding is not
appropriate.

Training of Auditory Memory

It has been customary to begin auditory training with nonverbal stimuli
on the grounds that one should progress from gross to fine discrimination.
The implications of the research reviewed in this paper indicate that the
concept of progression from nonverbal to verbal stimuli is inappropriate
since the perception and recall of verbal and nonverbal material involve
different processes (Kimura, 1967; Liberman *et al.*, 1967; A.H. Ling,
1972). It has been demonstrated that hearing-impaired subjects are unable
to benefit substantially from the low frequency cues provided by the

transposition of high frequencies (D. Ling, 1969). This may have been because the cues were insufficiently like speech.

Hearing-impaired children encounter probems at each stage of memory processing: the auditory information entering the sensory store is often indistinct or distorted, abnormal coding and rehearsal strategies may be adopted in working memory and inadequate information may be transferred into the long-term memory store. Training is required at every stage.

Programmed instruction in the auditory discrimination of words had yielded dramatic gains within the training situation (e.g. Ling and Doehring, 1969; Doehring and Ling, 1971), even in subjects who have worn hearing aids and received auditory training as part of their education. Auditory training typically involves same/different judgments or identification of a stimulus from a set of several alternatives. Such training has severe limitations in that subjects are not required to make categorical judgments about the stimuli and subsequently may be unable to identify them when they occur in other contexts. Hearing-impaired children should therefore receive training specifically to help them process long linguistic sequences. Such an ability is critical in reading. In order to comprehend a sentence, one has to be able to retain relevant information about the first part of the sentence while reading the latter part, likewise for a paragraph or a book. Verbatim memory is not required. A good reader is able to extract the meaning (semantic content) and store this as a *chunk*. His verbal skill enables him to reconstruct the story at a later date (Slobin, 1971).

In conclusion, if the aim of auditory training is to develop perceptual and memory skills which will promote the acquisition of normal speech and language patterns, it would seem important to provide graduated practice with speech material presented at a normal speaking rate. Furthermore, if experience with verbal sequences is provided, it should be possible for hearing-impaired children to develop a long-term memory store relating to the probabilities of phonological sequences occurring in English. Such knowledge has been shown to be important in the recall of verbal material (Broadbent, 1971).

REFERENCES

Aaronson, D.: Temporal factors in perception and short-term memory. *Psychol Bull,* 67:130–144, 1967.

Aaronson, D.: Temporal course of perception in an immediate recall task. *J Exp Psychol,* 76:129–140, 1968.

Affolter, F.D.: Developmental Aspects of Auditory and Visual Perception: An Experimental Investigation of Central Mechanisms of Auditory and Visual Processing. Unpublished doctoral dissertation. Pennsylvania State University, 1970.

Aten, J. and Davis, J.: Disturbances in the perception of auditory sequence in children with minimal cerebral dysfunction. *J Speech Hear Res* 11:236–245, 1968.

Atkinson, R.C. and Shiffrin, R.M.: The control of short-term memory. *Scientific American*, 225:82–90, 1971.

Blair, F.X.: A study of the visual memory of deaf and hearing children. *Am Ann Deaf*, 102:254–263, 1957.

Brill, R.G. and Orman, J.N.: An experiment in the training of deaf children in memory span for sentences. *Am Ann Deaf*, 98:270–279, 1953.

Broadbent, D.E.: The role of auditory localization in attention and memory span. *J Exp Psychol*, 47:191–196, 1954.

Broadbent, D.E.: *Decision and Stress.* New York: Academic Press, 1971.

Cole, R.A., Sales, B.D. and Haber, R.N.: Mechanisms of aural encoding: II The role of distinctive features in articulation and rehearsal. *Percept Psychophysics*, 6:343–348, 1969.

Conrad, R.: Acoustic confusions in immediate memory. *Brit J Psychol*, 55:75–84, 1964.

Conrad, R.: Short-term memory processes in the deaf. *Brit J Psychol*, 61:179–195, 1970.

Craik, F.I.M.: Primary memory. *British Medical Bulletin*, 27:232–236, 1971.

Crowder, R.G. and Morton, J.: Precategorical acoustic storage (PAS). *Percept Psychophysics*, 5.365–373, 1969.

DiFrancesca, K.B.: Recall of Visual Materials Presented Sequentially and Simultaneously by Deaf and Hearing Children. Unpublished doctoral dissertation. St. Louis University, 1969.

Doehring, D.G. and Ling, D.: Programmed instruction of hearing-impaired children in the auditory discrimination of vowels. *J Speech Hear Res*, 14:746–754, 1971.

Ebbin, J.B. and Edwards, A.E.: Speech sound discrimination of aphasics when intersound interval is varied. *J Speech Hear Res*, 10:120–125, 1967.

Fay, W.H.: *Temporal Sequence in the Perception of Speech.* Janua Linguarum, Nr. 45. The Hague: Mouton and Co., 1966.

Furth, H.G. and Pufall, P.B.: Visual and auditory sequence learning in hearing-impaired children. *J Speech Hear Res*, 9:441–449, 1966.

Furth, H.G. and Youniss, J.: Cognitive Structures Related to Verbal Deficiencies. Final Report RD–1484–S, Division of Research and Demonstration Grants, Social and Rehabilitation Service, Department of Health, Education and Welfare, Washington, D.C., 1969.

Gibson, J.J.: *The Senses as Perceptual Systems.* Boston: Houghton Mifflin Co., 1966.

Goetzinger, C.P. and Huber, T.G.: A study of immediate and delayed visual retention with deaf and hearing adolescents. *Am Ann Deaf*, 109:293–305, 1964.

Goodglass, H., Berko-Gleason, J. and Hyde, M.R.: Some dimensions of auditory language comprehension in aphasia. *J Speech Hear Res*, 13:595–606, 1970.

Hartung, J.E.: Visual perceptual skill, reading ability and the young deaf child. *Exceptional Children*, 36:603–608, 1970.

Hirsh, I.J.: Auditory perception of temporal order. *J Acoust Soc Am*, 31:759–767, 1959.

Kimura, D.: Some effects of temporal-lobe damage on auditory perception. *Canad J Psychol*, 15:156–165, 1961a.

Kimura, D.: Cerebral dominance and the perception of verbal stimuli. *Canad J Psychol*, 15:166–171, 1961b.

Kimura, D.: Left-right differences in the perception of melodies. *Quart J Exp Psychol*, XVI:355–358, 1964.

Kimura, D.: Functional asymmetry of the brain in dichotic listening. *Cortex*, 3:163–178, 1967.

Liberman, A.M., Cooper, F.S., Shankweiler, D.P. and Studdert-Kennedy, M.: Perception of the speech code. *Psychol Rev, 74:*431–461, 1967.

Ling, A.H.: Dichotic listening in hearing-impaired children. *J Speech Hear Res, 14:*793–803, 1971.

Ling, A.H.: Identification of Auditory Sequences by Hearing-Impaired and Normal-Hearing Children. Unpublished doctoral dissertation. McGill University, 1972.

Ling, D.: Speech discrimination by profoundly deaf children using linear and coding amplifiers. *I.E.E.E. Transactions on Audio and Electroacoustics, Vol. AU-17:*298–303, 1960.

Ling, D.: Implications of hearing aid amplification below 300 cps. *Volta Rev, 66:*723–729, 1964.

Ling, D. and Doehring, D.G.: Learning limits of deaf children for coded speech. *J Speech Hear Res, 12:*83–94, 1969.

Massaro, D.W.: Perceptual processes and forgetting in memory tasks. *Psychol Rev, 77:*557–567, 1970.

Milner, B.: Laterality effects in audition. In Mountcastle, V.B. (Ed.): *Interhemispheric Relations and Cerebral Dominance.* Baltimore: Johns Hopkins University Press, 1962, pp. 177–195.

Neisser, U.: *Cognitive Psychology.* New York: Appleton Century Crofts, 1967.

Norman, D.A. (Ed): *Models of Human Memory.* New York: Academic Press, 1970.

O'Connor, N. and Hermelin, B.: Spatial or Temporal Organisation of Memory? Unpublished manuscript, 1972.

Odom, P.B. and Blanton, R.L.: Phrase-learning in deaf and hearing subjects. *J Speech Hear Res, 10:*600–605, 1967.

Olsson, J.E. and Furth, H.G.: Visual memory-span in the deaf. *Am J Psychol, 79:*480–484, 1966.

Pintner, R. and Paterson, D.G.: A comparison of deaf and hearing children in visual memory for digits. *J Exp Psychol, 2:*76–88, 1917.   )

Powell, C.A.: Visual recognition in profoundly deaf children. *Sound, 5:*15–20, 1971.

Rosenthal, W.S.: Perception of Auditory Temporal Order as a Function of Selected Stimulus Features in a Group of Aphasic Children. Unpublished doctoral dissertation. Stanford University, 1970.

Ross, B.M.: Sequential visual memory and the limited magic of the number seven. *J Exp Psychol, 80:*339–347, 1969.

Shankweiler, D. and Studdert-Kennedy, M.: Identification of consonants and vowels presented to left and right ears. *Quart J Exp Psychol, 19:*59–63, 1967.

Shulman, H.G.: Similarity effects in short-term memory. *Psychol Bull, 75:*399–415, 1971.

Slobin, D.I.: *Psycholinguistics.* Glenview: Scott, Foresman and Co., 1971.

Sperling, G.A.: The information available in brief visual presentations. *Psychological Monographs, 74,* 1960. Whole No. 498.

Sperling, G.A.: A model for visual memory tasks. *Hum. Factors, 5:*17–31, 1963.

Studdert-Kennedy, M. and Shankweiler, D.: Hemispheric specialization for speech perception. *J Acoust Soc Am 48:*579–594, 1970.

Thomas, I.B., Hill, P.B., Carroll, F.S. and Garcia, B.: Temporal order in the perception of vowels. *J Acoust Soc Am 48:*1010–1013, 1970.

Warren, R.M. and Obusek, C.J.: Identification of temporal order within auditory sequences. *Percept Psychophysics, 12:*86–90, 1972.

Warren, R.M., Obusek, C.J., Farmer, R.M. and Warren, R.P.: Auditory sequence: Confusion of patterns other than speech or music. *Science, 164:*586–587, 1969.

Warren, R.M. and Warren, R.P.: Auditory illusions and confusions. *Scientific American,* 223:30–36, 1970.

White, C.T. and Cheatham, P.G.: Temporal numerosity: IV A comparison of the major senses. *J Exp Psychol,* 58:441–444, 1959.

Winitz, H.L.: *Articulatory Acquisition and Behavior.* New York: Appleton Century Crofts, 1969.

Withrow, F.B.: Immediate memory span of deaf and normally-hearing children. *Exceptional Children,* Sept. 1968, 33–41.

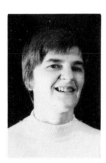

AGNES H. LING, Ph.D.

Agnes H. Ling was born in Newmains, Scotland. She was educated at Newmains School and Hamilton Academy and received her M.A. Degree from Glasgow University in 1953, her Diploma in Education of the Deaf from Manchester University in 1954 and her teaching certificate from Jordanhill Training College, Glasgow in 1954.

Dr. Ling was Assistant Teacher, Donaldson's School for the Deaf, Edinburgh, 1955–57; assistant teacher, special class for deaf children, Reading, England full time, 1957–60, part-time 1961–63; guidance service for parents of deaf babies, Montreal 1963–69; senior research assistant, McGill University Projects for Deaf Children, 1966–69 and M. Sc. degree in Human Communication Disorders, 1970.

Dr. Ling is married with two sons, aged 10 and 12 years.

Chapter XIII

THE AUDITORY APPROACH IN MEXICO
THROUGH O.I.R.A.

ENELDA LUTTMANN

I<small>T</small> <small>IS</small> <small>OBVIOUS</small> why the Auditory, Unisensory approach is so readily rejected. The simplicity of resorting primarily and expressly to the need to learn to hear, to learn to identify the sounds that are heard and apply the speech sounds to meaningful situations and to thought and development of ideas seems far too simple, seems far too similar to the steps employed by the non-deaf child who spontaneously acquires speech through the same procedure, and therefore, as he has his hearing, is expected to do so. But obviously, most people say, it is crazy to believe a child without hearing can hear. Perhaps, they say, with the use of hearing aids, he can distinguish the drum, the bell, but it is beyond reason to feel he could ever hear the parts of speech or develop all the complex knowledge involved in understanding language and the syntax of speech through hearing. They forget, or do not know, the steps of development that the hearing child has to go through—that the first year of life is that of learning to listen and identify sounds, is the practice of babbling, of hearing his own voice, of the constant chatter from his mother as she happily talks about everyday activities related to the child—such as the water being too hot for his bath, let's put in some cold, without expecting him to understand or answer. She talks, and he babbles back, and she laughs and shows great pleasure at his prespeech sounds. Then once spoken words start to appear, they forget the hearing child follows definite steps of development, has difficulty pronouncing certain sounds, leaves out certain phonemes, does not use pronouns or conjuctives until a certain age. In other words, they are not acquainted with, or conscious of, all the normal steps of development covered by a nondeaf child as he develops language and utters speech sounds and gets stuck pronouncing certain words with blends of consonants, etc. Or if they do know, they see no relationship with what a two-year-old with hearing is doing and what a four- or five-year-old deaf child is accomplishing after two or three years of auditory work.

107

They forget this deaf child was born to sound two years ago and must receive all those experiences that a hearing child gets; they forget to associate what a nondeaf child has accomplished after two or three years of auditory work.

Too easily, excuses are made and found, presupposed statements are issued: "He is too deaf to respond at this distance or that," "He is too deaf to hear those high frequency sounds," "It is impossible for him to hear the 'S' phoneme or the high frequency phonemes." But some deaf children, given half the chance, have taken us by surprise if we have faith in what they can do.

Some people are scientifically proving of late why a deaf child can do what a few people who took the patience, the time and effort to teach and expect accomplishment have known can be achieved. At first it was believed to exist in only a few, isolated cases, freaks or because one individual had taken pains to work with a very bright child—the results were exceptional but not to be expected for all children. The general outlook was, and still is, pessimistic.

Do we in normal conditions analyze the forms of speech or expect to be able to speak or learn another language? When we are learning something, do we have to rationalize how we learn, how we think in order to learn? Unless they are particularly interested in studying this human function, most people put their energies into learning the subject of their choice, be it physics, chemistry, biology, mathematics, engineering, music or any of the innumerable choices offered in this world of today, without a thought as to why they are capacitated to do so or how they will do it. Nobody insists on a previous study of their brain patterns, mental capacities or their motor coordination or any possible deviation from the norm. It is not looked for, and if it exists, not even noticed. How many examples do we have of famous or successful people who have achieved much in a particular specialty and yet if known at closer range have some imperfection, be it character, personality or physical, which has not detracted from their capacity to become outstanding.

Yet with a deaf child, or any other child with a handicap, one is immediately anxiously, tensely observing the child, noticing his differences, expecting him not to be able to function and expecting and looking for negative qualities and additional handicaps.

I remember so clearly when I first learned my child was deaf and knew nothing about what this entailed and decided to find out. First I found that many people who worked with the deaf covered their activities with a cloak of secrecy. I was told I could not comprehend, it was far too complex a problem, and unless I made up my mind to take a long and intensive course, I could not communicate with these specialists, be it teacher of the deaf, a speech therapist or what have you. On inquiring what, where and how I could learn and study, I found no information could be imparted. For a while, I was made to feel like a brainless dimwit. No matter what I had accomplished during my life time, nothing, but nothing, could help me grasp or understand the problem of deafness in order to help my own child.

I was supposed to accept this dreadful, mysterious affliction that had affected my son; yet, I could do little but hope that my boy might grow up to be mildly pleasant, moderately sociable, learn to live with rebuffs from others because of his lack of communication and to live with the idea that he could not talk and could not make himself understood, except in very limited situations. This prognosis was offered only if I handed him over, lock, stock and barrel, to a bunch of supernatural individuals with whom he would live during most of his formative years. If I asked what was to be achieved, why these particular methods should achieve these results or even if there was any proof that any results could be obtained, I never received an explanatory answer, at least not enlightening or comprehensive to my mentality. I could not grasp the reasons or be given positive assurance as to the methods employed and why they were employed; and yet, all these difficult and complex activities which they found too hard to explain to me were supposed to help a small, deaf boy become a useful citizen of the world he lived in, in spite of living in an unnatural, isolated environment, away from his home and family during the crucial learning period of his life.

Being a layman, being only a mother of a deaf child, my only source of judgment was seeing other deaf children at different stages of their development and observing what they had accomplished and achieved during childhood, preadolescence, adolescence and adulthood. Then I really did become depressed, for the more I looked, the more bewildered I became. It seemed so incredible that with all the advances in science, in knowledge of human function, mental and physical, so little was known about deafness, and few people with creative minds or rational thinking were involved. I became so tired of the same cliches and felt as if I had awakened into a world of fanatical beings who had been given religiously and systematically half-baked ideas with little logical background. But because someone 150 years ago had come up with what they thought was the solution for giving the deaf some form of communication, this method was still in its totality applicable in this day and age without modifications. These people, or specialists, had been taught to memorize and to do but not to think and create and never to query.

Later I learned there had been some variances in ideas and some pioneering work had evolved but had been all too easily lost and swallowed up and probably squashed from existence by the vested interests and lazy thinking of the majority.

During the time I was investigating about the work with the deaf, and as a result of indications from the Alexander Graham Bell Institute in Washington, I headed for Los Angeles and the John Tracy Clinic. Their evaluation of my boy fitted into the previous prognosis, but their guidance started earlier, at two years instead of four as indicated by the schools of the deaf, and they did offer parent guidance and explanations as to the meaning of deafness and all it implied. I had still to wait a year before any active attitude or constructive work could be carried out. I was told "No hearing available," but talk to the child I must, with my face in the light, etc. At that time, they had a complicated set of equipment in the basement, basically an electroencephalographic device, but unfortuately the results achieved from this impressive machinery did not offer any further information.

I had the great fortune of meeting Dr. Boris Morkovin and Miss Lucilla Moore at about this time, now twelve years ago. Dr. Morkovin developed a fatherly interest in this distressed and distraught mother, had long talks with me, imparted much information and knowledge and introduced me to everyone he thought worthwhile, either physically if distance permitted or through reading, over a period of years before his death. I would listen to him, and we would think out loud together. I learned to begin to understand what deafness was and learned what people were doing.

Actually after my second trip to Los Angeles, I bought an Auditory Training Unit, contrary to professional advice, since the general consensus was that my child had no usable hearing. He was profoundly deaf, and I was to accept that he had to learn to develop his other senses in compensatory degrees. But through using the trainer, he did respond after one-and-one-half years of amplified sound. Though sound had no meaning for him yet, I became convinced that he could hear something. I wrote excited and enthusiastically to Dr. Morkovin, feeling very strongly that my son had residual hearing and that it should be put to use and not neglected.

I went to Houston to the Speech and Hearing Clinic and saw that children were being fitted with hearing aids in one ear and parents shown to work accordingly. Specialized teachers worked with small groups of children one-half to one hour daily, with parents watching through a Gessell mirror. They started with deaf youngsters at one-and-one-half years! Unfortunately, I had not taken my child with me at that time.

After communicating with Dr. Morkovin and through his recommendation, that same year in May, I went to Los Angeles and met Dr. Ciwa Griffiths and saw the work at the HEAR Foundation. Before going, I had received and read their literature describing their approach and ideas. I had to hold myself in check and not get too excited until I saw in person what it was all about.

After spending a week with Dr. Griffiths and having her fit my son binaurally with hearing aids when he was two years and eight months old and learning as much as I could about the work they were doing, I managed to arrange to have Dr. Griffiths and Mrs. Betty Pettersen come to Mexico City early in July because I was convinced that they were on the right track.

In Mexico, Dr. Griffiths gave talks to a public gathered through notices in the paper, with a few parents of deaf children whom I had already met. She was scoffed by the existing oral school in our city. In October 1962, we opened O.I.R.A. with the help of four teachers trained by Dr. Griffiths at HEAR and Occidental College and a handful of deaf children, seven in total with their six pairs of parents.

While Dr. Griffiths worked with our first four teachers during the summer and fall months of 1962, I managed to meet Dr. Huizing in Gronningen, Holland, and Miss Edith Whetnall and her staff at the Audiology Unit of the Royal National Nose, Throat and Ear Hospital on Grays Inn Road. Here I spent two weeks meeting and talking and learning, with the utmost collaboration and great patience and time given by all those I came in contact with. All were ready to explain fully, physicians as well as teaching staff and parents. I encountered the same outstanding collaboration that I had received previously at HEAR Foundation. Nothing was too bothersome to explain, no questions too foolish to answer, and the rationality of the viewpoints presented was confirmed by the results of the children I met.

I wrote to Hallowell Davis whom I had previously contacted by mail and told him of my decision to work with my son on the auditory basis as practised by Dr. Griffiths and Miss Whetnall. He congratulated me on my decision and informed me that he knew of their work and admired it and had also concluded that the auditory approach or method applied at early ages was considered the indicated procedure. This occurred in 1962 before the International Congress for the Education of the Deaf was held in Washington in July 1963. I was shocked to meet many people from C.I.D. whose general attitude or approach did not indicate Hallowell Davis's criteria had had much effect at that date. Unfortunately, I personally have not been in contact with C.I.D. of late, but in Mexico City I did meet at the Audiology Congress some of the staff and found very young children that were being worked with but not with a true auditory approach—that of living in a normal environment with family cooperation and guidance in the handling of the auditory work for the development of speech and language through hearing—which I deem so necessary for a true unisensory emphasis.

While assisting the International Congress for the Education of the Deaf in Washington in 1963, I had the privilege of meeting Dr. Daniel Ling. I had been particularly interested in Guberinas presentation and ideas and was told by Michael Reed that Dr. Ling was well acquainted with his work in Paris. After long talks and discussions, Dr. Ling accepted an invitation to come to Mexico and to become a Consultant Director, as were Dr. Griffiths and Miss Whetnall, who had spent very productive and eye-opening weeks on different occasions, working intensely with us in Mexico. They also continuously sent us pertinent information or advice through the mail.

Both Drs. Agnes and Daniel Ling have made frequent, short-term visits to Mexico, complete with intensive work, which has been of invaluable and incomparable help in the development of the work with our deaf children at O.I.R.A.

Dr. L. Fisch, whose work at the Heston Clinic in London and the Nuffield Speech and Hearing Center in the same city is outstanding, has also given generously of his time and knowledge.

In my own personal experience as Director (functioning part time, sharing duties as wife, mother of three very active hearing children and one deaf 13-year-old, as President of the Board of O.I.R.A. and coordinating the activities of the auditory teaching of our deaf children and the guiding of their mothers and fathers, I find two outstanding factors keep looming: a constant slackening of parent guidance and of real auditory work, which I consider are the bases for teaching speech and language through the unisensory approach and utilizing the hearing with wide range amplification.

We are a parent-oriented center. Our parent has to personally assist and participate actively in the specialized auditory individual—one child, teacher, parent class. The child is generally assisted twice a week. Obviously, this period of time would be useless if the parent was not expected to carry on the work at home during the everyday experiences with the child in his waking hours.

We primarily employ school teachers with either kindergarten or primary school training, preferably with two years of experience in teaching normal, nondeaf children. We give them a specialized course on teaching a deaf child to speak, using the auditory approach with wide-range amplification, and we call ourselves a parent-guidance center.

As the teachers, especially the primary school teachers, are originally trained to work with the child, to teach him his ABC's, reading, writing, arithmetic and other scholastic subjects, one has to watch that these subjects do not infiltrate and overtake the importance of work with language and speech production and all the nuance of pitch, articulation, rhythm and stress. Then again, in our concern for developing vocabulary, spoken and comprehensive language, with correct syntax, we have to be careful that we do not forget the fluidity and quality of voice. We must constantly be reminding the deaf child to use his hearing for understanding speech and language. We must constantly remember to check how much the child is hearing, irrespective of what the audiogram demonstrates he cannot hear. We must constantly ask ourselves if we have given him the best audibility, or if we can do better.

It is essential to keep in mind the equivalent steps of development of a normal hearing child and not jump too soon into artificial, unnatural methods of correcting voice quality or articulation in a deaf child. It is all too easy to resort too soon to other methods of teaching speech and language correction other than through hearing. Other methods should be used as a last resort. They should only be employed initially for the child to grasp what you want him to do and then withdrawn. The instructor should refrain from further tactile or visual methods, reminding the child which is the correct pattern through voice and hearing only.

It is essential to conscientiously test how and what the child is hearing, the functioning of his hearing aids and if there is any conductive overlay. With the ever-improving electronic knowledge and better amplification, such as the Electrex microphone, there will be less excuse to use anything other than the Auditory Trainer or Individual Aids for production of speech and language.

Our aim is to prepare a deaf child so that he can attend a normal hearing school on the basis of one deaf child per classroom of hearing children. We recommend that they start at the age of three in a normal pre-kindergarten. We have found that the majority of our children require additional scholastic help once formal primary school work has started. In some cases, the mother can cope on her own, with guidance and help from the center. When the child needs further help, we employ various methods. The most common method consists of after-school, group classes at the center with scholastic assistance and reinforcement of relevant vocabulary, in addition to the individual auditory work. At times we have had a specialized auditory teacher attend a school where various children attend. Occasionally it has been necessary to take a child from the regular classroom for a limited period of time for special school work until we feel that the child has overcome his difficulties and can return to a normal school environment full time. The work with each child is varied according to their requirements, to the physical possibilities of distance, available teachers, numbers of children involved and economic capacity. But we definitely feel that we have failed if a child has come to us at infant or preschool age and is unable to attend a regular school and then has to attend a school for the deaf when he reaches school age.

Parental guidance and parental participation keep slackening. We have always insisted that the child should not be received in his individual, specialized class unless the parent also assists and is willing to collaborate and work at home. Obviously the two hours a week that the majority of children attend our center is useless unless the parent is constantly aware of opportunities throughout the day, whereby she can develop language and motivate and interest the child in a give-and-take of verbal communication. In practice, one too often sees the parent sitting taut and nervous and isolated—present physically but mentally distant. Unless the teacher conscientiously makes sure that the mother participates actively, we will never know how much attention is focused on the class. Nor will it be known how well the mother is relating to the child and if she has grasped the fundamental aspects of the particular activity being demonstrated.

The other problem which presents itself is that as the teachers develop assurance and personal pride in what they can do and achieve, they wish to prove what they are personally able to do and what they can accomplish with the deaf child. As they have originally been child-oriented in their regular teacher training course, they all too easily tend to leave out the parent. I believe that we should employ parents of successful, older deaf children, not having necessary teacher's degrees.

Many parents have shopped around, prior to coming to us and have been told conflicting ideas: "Your child is not deaf"; "He is non-educable"; "Mongoloid"; "Neurologically handicapped"; "Has central nervous disorders"; "Is aphasic"; "Put him into an institution for the mentally retarded or slow learners"; or have been told "Your child is too deaf, has no usable hearing, put him into an institution for the deaf." Or the other extreme: "He is a slow talker, he will develop on his own later; don't fret and worry." It makes my blood boil to still hear doctors issuing these same statements which I received twelve years ago to other parents.

It is obvious the parents cannot help being confused, undecided and afraid, trying to convince themselves that the doctors and professionals must be right, and yet seeing they cannot agree among themselves. When the mother arrives at a center with an auditory approach, she is still too emotionally worked up to do anything by herself. She appears indifferent, but in reality she is afraid of showing how much she does care and is afraid to breakdown.

When the teacher begins working on the methods employed to develop hearing and speech and language through everyday activities, the teacher must consciously create situations in the classroom where the child and the mother come in close contact. This will help the mother employ her pentup tensions by actively participating with the teacher and will in turn help the mother when on her own with her child.

It is so difficult for any human to remain aloof and cold with her own, small child next to her, putting his arms around her neck and kissing her, with friendly suggestions from the teacher as to how to incorporate language and speech sounds into everyday activities—or when sitting on the floor and playing ball and laughing and commenting and talking about it and being kissed and hugged throughout the game.

The teacher has to help the mother regain her self-esteem and self-confidence so that she recognizes that she can and must help her child. She is assured that she will share the responsibility with a team of medical, technical and teaching staffs and will receive the guidance and help from the center with the required modifications of activities in accordance to the child's development and needs.

In continuation, I will list some of the activities that we consider helpful in carrying out an appropriate family guidance program.

In effect, the mother is usually the only individual who deals with the rehabilitation on a regular basis, and the burden on her shoulders is often too much for her to cope with. We have found that if the center makes a point of asking the father to attend in person, inviting him to participate in his child's class once a month, his interest and understanding of the child and his difficulties become a positive factor, and he may even participate more often. Some fathers spontaneously attend weekly. The net result in the advancement of the child and the family relationship as a whole is immeasurable.

We also feel that it is necessary to encourage friendships among the parents and ask them to visit each other in their homes. Orientation is given to a mother who has been attending the center about a new arrival in terms of ways she could help and guide the newcomer in her own home environment. Definite guidance steps are discussed, but the approach is left up to the parent's initiative with a petition that she report her findings and activities to the teacher in charge of the new child and family. This information may be of help in organizing the program of work for this individual child by taking into consideration the home environment and family as seen through the visiting mother's eyes.

We have developed group meetings for the siblings of the deaf children directed by one of the teachers of the center; the purpose is for them to meet each other and freely voice their feelings, share their frustrations and complaints and thereby ease the tensions developed by jealousies or guilt feelings in their relationship with their handicapped siblings. For example, an older brother can feel responsible for the deafness of the younger because at his birth, he felt displaced, resented the competition and attention the baby received and perhaps wished him harm, or even death, anything to do away with him and regain the parents full, unshared attention. Much insight has developed from these groups for the youngsters and adults. We have worked with small groups of 10 to 15 children between the approximate ages of 6–8, 9–11, 12–15 years.

Group meetings are held every fifteen days, each teacher with her particular set of parents, where she can reinforce basic topics—such as knowledge of the functioning of the hearing aids, interpretation of audiograms, language development—with the steps followed by a nondeaf child and where the parents can discuss their particular children in the development ladder and where the children are heading.

Monthly meetings are called for all parents, adult family members and teachers, with organized, alternate months when lectures or special programs are presented by the parents and by the teachers.

Introductory talks are given by the head teachers to small groups of parents who recently entered the center on the meaning of hearing and deafness, how speech develops, the role of the parent in the program and other pertinent points. These are done with a simple and clear presentation for better understanding of the deaf child and his handicap, the negative and positive factors, with marked emphasis on proper audibility and guidance.

Eventual social programs are organized for specific events such as Mother's Day, Children's Day, Teacher's Day or excursions to the country, fairs, etc. These social events are very important in order to break away from the formal instructive, conscientiously-guided meetings where the relationship between parents is focused on the deaf child, his requirements, their participation and cooperation.

Occasionally, small groups of parents are stimulated to get together informally in each other's home, where more intimate friendships can develop in order that they can share, understand and help each other. It must be mentioned that apart from these group activities, a parent is always free to ask for and obtain a private interview with the director, the head teacher, the coordinating head teachers, the psychologist or the medical audiologist. These coordinating teachers are constantly observing the classes through the Gessell mirrors that give visual and auditory access to each individual classroom without interrupting the class or the participants being conscious of the observation. We feel it very beneficial that each working teacher be given the benefit of sporadic, constructive observation and evaluation of the work being carried out. These observation rooms are indispensable for teaching parents or new personnel.

Quite separate from our regular children that live in Mexico City, we have always attended a large number of children. that live throughout the republic and some in other Latin American countries.

When an out-of-town parent arrives with their child, they attend specialized, one-hour classes daily with child and teacher. Extra orientation and guidance is given to the parent alone; they are required to remain a minimum of ten days.

An evaluation of the child is made upon arrival. A diagnostic study is carried out covering an audiological, pediatric and E.N.T. evaluation, as well as a psychological one, indicating the maturation levels of development—motor, language and social.

The out-of-town parent learns what her role is. Her program of work for the next three months is explained and demonstrated. Each program is patterned on a particular child and his necessities and developed according to his personal requirements—taking into account age, hearing loss, social, economic and educational level of the family. Upon termination of this ten-day period, the parent leaves with a clear and simple basic plan of work which she will report to us by correspondence as she proceeds to carry it out. The parent and child are required to return at least twice during the year for a week's stay. Recently Mrs. Barbara Rushmer, a teacher of the deaf in Nassau, Bahamas, gave me the idea of using tape recorders and cassettes, which we plan to employ at the earliest possible opportunity. How much easier to explain and demonstrate with them than through long, written instruction. The mother can send us a taped sample of her methods of work with her child.

We are responsible for the formation of an Auditory Center in Merida, Yucatan, started by a group of four families with deaf children. This Center, in combination with the local government, handles approximately 60 children. Another center was formed in Guadalajara, Jalisco, with about 45 to 50 children, and a small auditory unit was installed as part of a larger, general rehabilitation in Toluca, Mexico, where two psychologists have been working with children of very low cultural and economic levels. Various individuals have come to take our teacher training course and have worked with us for awhile with the aim of starting work in their own location. We have had teachers from various Latin American countries, such as Panama, San Salvador, Colombia, Uruguay, Venezuela and others, all of whom return with an auditory approach for working with deaf children in their home countries.

Far too slowly perhaps but definitely, the auditory approach towards work with deaf children is being employed and is extending further afield. Let us hope we will see a very marked increase.

ENELDA LUTTMANN, B.A.

Mrs. Luttmann received her primary education in England and her high school was completed after her arrival in Mexico, receiving her Bachelor of Arts Degree from Texas University. Mrs. Luttmann's work at Texas University was in the premedical field, with a minor in psychology and social studies placing an emphasis on child development.

She first became interested in work with the deaf in 1960 when she began to suspect her son, Ricky, was experiencing hearing difficulties. Ricky was first fitted with aids at the HEAR Foundation, Pasadena, in 1961. Her interest in work with her own son led to the founding of O.I.R.A. (Orientation Infantil Para Rehabilatacion Audiologica, A.C.) in Mexico by Mr. and Mrs. Juan Luttmann in 1962, patterned after HEAR Foundation. This center has grown to the point where it is widely recognized throughout all of Mexico.

Chapter XIV

A SCHOOL SYSTEM ADOPTS
THE AUDITORY APPROACH IN FLORIDA

Robert Wieland

Broward County Public Schools adopted HEAR Foundation techniques in 1967. At that time, one therapist serviced ten children, several of whom had been initially evaluated at HEAR Foundation in California. Each child was scheduled for therapy on a twice weekly basis and was given intensive auditory training. Each child in the program was also enrolled in a school with hearing children; thus, each child was supplied with individualized auditory training and language experiences, as well as a normal hearing environment.

SALT (Specialized Auditory and Language Training) Program is the name we have given to our public school clinical program for the hearing-impaired. Teachers in the SALT Program are certified in speech pathology, audiology and/or deaf education. We now have four, full-time teachers who service 36 children. The children range in age from two to 14 years. Certain changes have evolved from the original HEAR Foundation format as the program has grown and because of the nature of a public school program.

Initially, all children were required to have binaural amplification. Although we strongly feel that this is the most appropriate type of amplification, we feel we cannot deprive a child of our services if a family is unable to provide binaural amplification. Over 85 percent of the children do have binaural fittings and benefit from them tremendously; however, it is no longer a requirement for enrollment in the program.

Initially, all children were scheduled for therapy twice a week. Now that our program has expanded, we are able to schedule more flexibly and thus better meet each child's individual needs. Many of our preschoolers are seen four times a week. Significant progress has been noted when therapy has been increased. A few of the older children are seen only once a week; four children between the ages of 8 and 12 have been dismissed because they no longer need therapy. Schedules vary with the child's needs, his school schedule and his parent's ability to provide transportation. Elementary school age children are scheduled early in the morning or late in the afternoon in an effort not to interrupt their academic studies and in order to make their school day as much like their peers as possible. Regular classroom teachers have been most cooperative in adjusting children's schedules for therapy, as they generally are for hearing children who need remedial reading or speech therapy.

The SALT Program is now able to enroll hearing-impaired children as soon as their loss is identified. Prior to acceptance in the program, all children must receive medical and audiological clearance. The school system does not have the equipment necessary for complete audiological evaluations, so the children are seen by the audiologist at the Easter Seal Clinic. This audiologist is also responsible for fittings of hearing aids. The school system does have three certified, clinical audiologists, and if at sometime in the future we acquire an audiological suite, audiological hearing aid evaluations could be done as part of the educational program.

The majority of a SALT therapist's time is spent with preschool children. These children are seen as often as four times a week. HEAR Foundation techniques for auditory training and language development are used. We use the HEAR Training Unit extensively, although we also work with the children with their own hearing aids on a regular basis. Therapy is aimed at making full use of the child's residual hearing. No formal speech-reading is taught, as the children seem to naturally acquire this on their own; language is never presented without voice. All lessons are taught initially in a face to face position, but then the therapist gradually moves to the side of the child and then behind him. Not every child can learn to make fine discriminations, but many can. Some of the profoundly deaf students can follow two-step commands that are spoken in a natural voice behind them. All students are taught to turn when their name is called; this is necessary for two reasons—one, as a safety measure and two, so that a teacher or parents can call a child and get his attention. (It makes for much less frustrating communication.)

We do not wait until a child has perfectly intelligible speech before we place him in a regular classroom. Many first graders have speech problems, a few are unintelligible; no one would keep a cleft palate child out of regular school just because he was difficult to understand. Intelligibility frequently improves dramatically when the child is motivated to communicate with his hearing peers.

Broward County has 120 deaf children. Over 50 percent of these children are in regular classes with their hearing peers. Seven self-contained, hearing-impaired classrooms are available for students unable to meet with success in the regular school program. Many of these students have additional handicaps or come to us with poor or inadequate early training.

The hearing-impaired child enrolled in the regular classroom is eligible for three types of supplementary services. Almost all children with severe and profound losses receive individualized auditory training and language development through the SALT Program. In addition, a hearing-impaired child who is achieving one year or more below grade level is eligible for the services of the academic tutors. We have five academic tutors covering different geographical sections of the county. The child is seen from one to four hours per week, depending upon his needs. The task of the academic tutor is to meet the child's specific academic needs. For example, if the regular classroom teacher presents a unit on evaporation and the hearing-impaired child does not fully understand the concept, the academic tutor reinforces and elaborates the first presentation. In other cases, academic tutors may help the child with vocabulary with which he is unfamiliar. The academic tutors provide a valuable liaison between the SALT therapists and the regular classroom teacher.

Another service for which the hearing-impaired child is eligible is speech therapy. Over 40 speech therapists service the hearing children in the public schools. Hearing-impaired students are scheduled as needed on either a group or individual basis. Many times, it is beneficial for the deaf child to be enrolled in a group speech therapy class with his hearing peers; the child then realizes that even students with normal hearing must work on their speech production.

Children in the hearing-impaired program also receive the services of our Diagnostic Center. Every two years, the Hiskey-Nebraska Test of Learning Aptitude is administered to children enrolled in the SALT Program. The information received from this test allows the therapists to work to the child's strengths and to alleviate his weaknesses.

We are in the process of developing formal test batteries to help us better assess the academic achievement of children enrolled in regular classes. At present, the children are tested in their regular schools with their peers. In some schools, however, achievement tests are administered with the use of tape recordings or over the public address system; naturally, this puts the hearing-impaired child at a definite disadvantage. In these instances, the academic tutors are allowed to administer the tests on an individual basis.

Recently, psychometrists from our Diagnostic Center have begun administering batteries of tests to help us determine appropriate grade placement. Some of the tests administered include the Frostig, Slingerland, Winter Haven, WISC and Wide Range Achievement Test, as well as informal evaluations. Results enable the SALT therapist, academic tutor and classroom teacher to have an objective measure of the child's achievement. Too often classroom teachers either overestimate or underestimate the child's progress. Some teachers feel that the child has made less progress than he actually has because of difficulty in communication or following directions. On the other hand, other teachers are so delighted that the deaf child can do anything that they give credit were it is not due. We ask that the teachers grade the children enrolled in regular classes as they would their other students. If the teacher would retain a hearing child with skills similar to the deaf child's, then the deaf child should be retained. There is a tendency among professionals in the field to feel that a deaf child is successful in a regular school only if he is making straight A's and working above grade level. We need to remember that not all hearing children work at grade level. Each child needs to be evaluated according to his ability.

Both academic tutors and therapists from SALT are available at the beginning of the school year, and throughout the year, to provide the regular classroom teacher with an orientation to the deaf child's special needs. As yet, no formal program for the regular classroom teachers has been developed, but this is something we intend to work on for next year. Presently, orientation is accomplished through teacher conferences and written handouts. Since academic tutors have regular contact with the classroom teachers, they can often catch problems in the early stages.

All of the new schools being built in the county are open schools. This has many implications, both positive and negative, for the deaf child. Open schools tend to be more noisy than self-contained classrooms; the deaf child must learn to separate important from unimportant auditory stimuli. The child has many teachers instead of one—more people who need to be educated about his special needs, more people with whom the child needs to learn to communicate. The open school demands more independence on the child's part. He must learn to follow a schedule and do a certain amount of independent study. These things are not necessarily negative. Open schools increase the child's contacts with his hearing peers; he is more apt to learn to work in small groups with his peers. The open school concept fosters more interaction among the children and less of the traditional teacher-to-pupil lecturing. Teaching in open schools is often done with a group of children sitting close to the teacher; gone are the traditional rows of desks. The deaf child can easily maneuver his position so that he can be close to the teacher. Finally, the open schools abound in media, much of it visual and beautifully suited for the hearing-impaired student.

We feel the SALT Program has demonstrated that a clinical auditory training program can be offered successfully through a public school system. There are several ways in which we intend to expand the program. The first expansion is in its first stage and is in the area of extending our services to children under three years. We have just recently begun this part of the program and are looking forward to serving more *under three's* as we acquire two additional therapists this year. Early identification and training should insure that even more of our students than the present 50 percent can be enrolled in regular hearing classes.

Another way we intend to expand the program is through increased emphasis on parent counseling. Since parents provide transportation to the program we are able to see them on a regular basis. Each child is scheduled for an hour of the therapist's time. Approximately 45 minutes are devoted to therapy and the remaining time is spent talking with parents and writing anecdotal records. Many parents that have preschoolers just beginning the program have only recently learned that their child is deaf; often they have no practical knowledge of hearing loss and its social, education and psychological implications. Although some counseling is attempted during the initial interview, we feel it is imperative that parents receive additional information and counseling on a regular basis. It is important that both parents be involved whenever possible. Our plans call for small group meetings with one or two therapists and several parents with children of approximately the same age. Implementation of this program will begin as soon as another teacher can be hired.

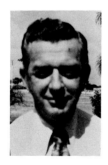

ROBERT G. WIELAND, Ed.D.

Dr. Wieland received his B.S. from Florida State University in 1952 majoring in Psychology. In 1953 he acquired his M.S. in the area of Child Clinical Psychology from the same university and received his doctorate in Education, majoring in Guidance and Counseling also from the University of Florida. He is certified as a Psychologist from the Florida State Board of Examiners. Dr. Wieland has had a wealth of experience in the following assignments: School Psychologist, Broward County Board of Public Instruction; Clinical Psychologist, parttime private practice in Broward County; Supervisor of Diagnostic and Clinical Services, Broward County Board of Public Instruction; Coordinator of Exceptional Child Program and Diagnostic and

Clinical Service and is presently Director of Exceptional Child Program, Diagnostic and Clinical Services and Related Services.

He is a member of the American Psychological Association, Division 16; Florida Psychological Association; Florida Education Association; Broward County Association of Deans and Counselors. He is a member of the advisory Board for Broward County Commission on Problems of Mental Health, Easter Seal Clinic, Broward Institute of Reading, United Cerebral Palsy and Vanguard School. Dr. Wieland is a member of the Board of Directors for Broward County Mental Health Association, Temple Beth El Nursery School and Kindergarten, Community Action Program, Easter Seal Clinic and Sun Dial School.

Chapter XV

INDIVIDUAL AUDITORY TRAINING SCHEMES IN REGULAR SCHOOLS

D.M.C. DALE

M OST OF THE work reported in providing auditory training and auditory experience for hearing-impaired children may be loosely classified into two main categories—graded listening exercises (Goldstein, 1939; Carhart, 1947; Huizing, 1951; Lowell and Stoner, 1960) and the full time use of hearing aids (Ewing, 1964; Watson, 1958; Whetnall and Fry, 1964). Before electronics were introduced into this field in the early 1930's, most emphasis was of necessity placed on the use of listening exercises; however, since the introduction of lightweight hearing aids, their fulltime use seems to have become an accepted aim for all but a handful of children.

There has been little scientific work published in the field of auditory training. This may have been due to the difficulty of providing more than one or two *listening* sessions each week and the relative lack of success of such infrequent auditory training. (The daily use of tape recorders and techniques such as the listening-reading-speaking method (Dale, 1971) seems, to the teachers concerned, to aid many children's speech discrimination, but unfortunately no statistics have been published to substantiate this.)

Recording and playback instruments such as *Language masters* appear to have the capacity to provide frequent auditory training sessions for individual children (Crane and Bollback Evans, 1962). After observing these instruments in use with aphasic children and with severely deaf teenagers, a preliminiary investigation was arranged to measure their effectiveness as aids to auditory training. One group of seven severely deaf children (M=97.43dB) and another of profoundly deaf (M=110.14dB) were selected. Mr. John Pym conducted the initial and final testing and supervised all practice sessions.

Forty sentences and phrases were used for both testing and training. These were arranged on ten cards, four per card, e.g. List 1:

a. The boy played football.
b. Hello Bobby.
c. The car went very fast.
d. Where are you going?

Both groups were tested at the beginning and end of the three-week period.

Group 1 had listening practice five minutes each day.
Group 2 had two sessions daily of ten minutes each,

The child was shown the first card of four sentences. He listened to each sentence as it was played through the language master, while the experimenter indicated the position of each syllable. He was allowed to listen to each phrase or sentence as often as he desired (sometimes this was five or six times). The remaining nine sets of four phrases and sentences were then presented in the same manner. Fourteen consecutive school days were used for this auditory training work between the initial and final tests.

The results (Tables XV-I and XV-II) indicate an improvement on the retest scores of both groups, but in the case of Group 1, this did not reach statistical significance. In the case of Group 2, however, there was a very significant difference between means [t(for unrelated sample) = 4.15 with 12 degrees of freedom (p<.001)]. The enthusiastic response to the training program of the children in Group 2 was a most encouraging feature of this investigation.

Despite the lack of refinement evident in the above design, this pilot study has provided sufficient evidence that frequent use of recording and playback instruments does aid severely deaf children in speech discrimination. It is intended therefore to pursue this work further with the following adaptations and checks:

1. Larger experimental and control groups will be matched as nearly as possible for age, intelligence, hearing loss and age of onset of deafness, language development and social background.
2. The effect of training will be measured to ascertain the degree, if any, of transfer of training to speech material which has not been specifically learned through auditory training.
3. The effect of more frequent training periods on profoundly deaf children (as included in Group 1) will be studied.
4. The effect of increased speech discrimination on the subjects' own speech production will be measured.
5. The practicability of introducing auditory training in schools and

Table XV-I

RESULTS OF FOURTEEN-DAY AUDITORY TRAINING

Group 1 Profoundly deaf children—One 5 minute training session per day

CHILD	HEARING ° LOSS	AGE	ONSET OF DEAFNESS	I.Q. TEACHERS' EST.	TEST 1	TEST 2	DIFF. BETWEEN SCORES
1.	112	10.2	BIRTH	C	6	11	+5
2.	115	10.2	"	C+	8	12	+4
3.	112	10.4	"	D	7	8	+1
4.	110	10.2	"	C+	5	8	+3
5.	100	9.11	"	C+	16	15	−1
6.	110	9.9	"	A	24	20	−4
7.	112	11.3	"	C	11	12	+1
MEAN	110.14	10.3 yr. S.D. ± 4.96 m		C+ (APPROX)	11.00	12.29	+1.29 NS

Table XV-II

RESULTS OF FOURTEEN-DAY AUDITORY TRAINING

Group 2 Severely deaf children—Two 10 minute training sessions per day

CHILD	HEARING LOSS*	AGE	ONSET OF DEAFNESS	I.Q. TEACHERS' EST.	TEST 1	TEST 2	DIFF. BETWEEN SCORES
8	98	8.1	BIRTH	C	6	29	+ 13
9	77	10.2	"	D	23	38	+ 15
10	110	9.3	"	C+	13	21	+ 8
11	102	8.4	"	B	10	24	+ 14
12	102	8.1	"	C+	8	23	+ 15
13	98	8.2	"	C−	11	25	+ 14
14	95	9.6	"	D+	4	15	+ 11
MEAN	97.43	8.10 yr. SD ± 8.62 m		C (APPROX)	10.71	25.00	+ 14.29 Highly Signif.

*Mean of 500, 1000, 2000 Hz in the better ear

classes for hearing-impaired children will be investigated, as well as in the individually integrated situation.

Individual integration is at present being studied in the Haringey Education Authority in North London. It was proposed that this project be mentioned at a forward-looking meeting such as this, since it seems to represent a possible break away from our conventional methods of teaching deaf and partially hearing children. It should provide splendid opportunities for individual participation not only in auditory training, but also in speech, language, reading and lipreading, as well as in social situations. (One factor which is felt to be educationally detrimental to deaf children (Department of Education and Science, 1964; *Education of the Deaf* 1965; Gentile and Di Francesca, 1969) is that, due largely to their low reading ages, individual work is difficult to arrange and numerous *whole class* lessons need to be conducted. It has been noted, however, that most hearing-impaired children respond well to individual teaching. A number of children, for example, who have been observed to speak only two or three times in 15 minutes during a group language lesson speak no less than 25 times in only five minutes when taught on a one-to-one basis.

Projected Research

It is intended to conduct an experiment with a group of six children aged nine and ten years who are to be withdrawn from a unit for partially hearing children in a regular school. We intend to enroll them in their own local schools, and each child will be assisted by an itinerant teacher of the deaf for up to 45 minutes each day. Each class teacher of the ordinary school will also help in the limited amount of time she has available. Each child will also have an assistant teacher (half-time) to help him interpret what is happening. Approximately two hours each day will be devoted to individual teaching.

We anticipate that *the teacher of deaf children* will:

a) give individual speech and language teaching to the hearing-impaired children every day
b) evaluate the previous day's programs attempted by the deaf children and construct new ones
c) liaise as closely as possible with the class teachers (and head teachers) on all aspects of the deaf children's educational and social development
d) guide and encourage the assistant teachers each day
e) visit the homes of the deaf children with the assistant teachers to hear their problems and give appropriate guidance

f) administer periodical audiological, educational and social adjustment tests to the children. (These will also be administered by the research workers.)

g) feel responsible for the deaf child's success or lack of it in the program.

The assistant teacher will be able to assist in a variety of ways, including the following:

a) devise and consolidate material presented by the class teacher

b) interpret information such as school or class announcements to ensure that the deaf child understands what is going on

c) by example and precept, encourage the normally hearing children to bring the handicapped child into group conversations and activities

d) under the general guidance and supervision of the teacher of the deaf children, set up apparatus for the individual programs in reading, language and auditory training, using film strips, slides, language master, tape recorder and 8mm cine loop films for lipreading practice

e) report, in very considerable detail, the events of each day to the parents

f) report daily to the teacher of the deaf.

Parents should, as suggested above, be given an unprecedented amount of information about their child's school day and will be encouraged to make the very most of this after school each day, but perhaps, more importantly, on future occasions when the material crops up in other meaningful natural situations.

Research measurements

Educational attainment tests (Hamp, 1970; Dale, 1971; Orwid, 1960; Spencer, 1971) have been administered twice last year. The same measures will be applied twice this year, and the velocity of each child's educational progress will be obtained in both situations. Audiological tests (Rutter, Tizard and Whitmore, 1970) and social adjustment ratings (Dale, 1970) have also been administered and will be repeated in 1973.

Observations will be made of the reactions of the deaf children, the normally hearing children, the parents of both groups, the teachers and assistant teachers.

If this scheme proves successful it is hoped to continue it and extend it to more severely handicapped children.

REFERENCES

Carhart, R.: Auditory Training. In Silverman, S.R., and Davis, H.: *Hearing and Deafness*. New York, Holt, Rinehart, and Winston Inc., 1947, p. 368.

Crane, N.W. and Bollback Evans, B.: A Talking Dictionary. *Volta Review, 64:* 1962.

Dale, D.M.C.: *Applied Audiology for Children*. Springfield, Thomas, 1970.

Dale, D.M.C.: *Deaf Children at Home and at School*. London: University of London Press, 1971, p. 222.

Department of Education and Science: *The Health of the School Child 1962 and 1963*. H.M.S.O., 1964.

Education of the Deaf. Report to the Secretary, Department of Health, Education and Welfare, Washington, D.C., 1965.

Ewing, A.W.G. and Ewing, E.C. *Teaching Deaf Children to Talk*. University of Manchester Press, 1964.

Gentile, A. and Di Francesca, S. *Academic Achievement Test Performance of Hearing Impaired Students* (National survey results). Washington, D.C.: 1969.

Goldstein, M.A.: *The Acoustic Method for Training of the Deaf or Hard of Hearing Child*. Laryngoscope Press, 1939.

Hamp, N.E.: *A Reading Vocabulary Picture Test for Deaf and Partially Hearing Children*. Unpublished M.Ed. Thesis. Leicester University Department of Education, 1970.

Huizing, H.: Auditory training. *Acta Otolaryng Supp, 100:*158–163, 1951.

Lowell, E. and Stoner, M.: *Play It by Ear*. Los Angeles: John Tracy Clinic, 1960.

Owrid, H.L.: Measuring spoken language in young deaf children. *The Teacher of the Deaf, 58:*Part 1:24–34; Part 2:124–128, 1960.

Rutter, M., Tizard, J. and Whitmore, K.: *Education, Health and Behavior*, Appendices 5 and 6. Longmans, 1970.

Spencer, L.M.: The Construction of a Test of the Intelligibility of the Speech of Deaf and Partially Hearing Children. Unpublished Ph.D. thesis. University of London Institute of Education, 1971.

Watson, T.J.: Some factors affecting the successful use of hearing aids by children. In Ewing, A.W.G. (Ed.): *The Modern Educational Treatment of Deafness*. University of Manchester Press, 1958, pp. 34/1–5.

Whetnall, E. and Fry, D.B.: *The Deaf Child*. Heinemann, 1964.

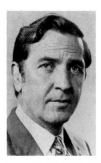

D.M.C. DALE, Ph.D.

Dr. Dale was born and educated in New Zealand. He received his B.A. and diploma in education from the University of Auckland and taught deaf children in New Zealand for five years.

After three years study under Professor Sir Alexander Ewing in Manchester University, he was awarded his Ph.D. and returned to New Zealand to lecture in the education of deaf children at Christchurch Teachers' College. In 1962 he was appointed principal of the School for Deaf Children, Auckland. In April 1965 he took up his present post as senior lecturer in Education of the Deaf at the University of London. His major research interest since 1960 has been in the field of integrating deaf children into regular schools. Dr. Dale has lectured in colleges and universities in the United States, Canada, Scandinavia and Australia.

He has written three books: *Applied Audiology for Children, Deaf Children at Home and at School* and *Language Development for Deaf Children*. Dr. Dale is married and has 2 children.

Chapter XVI

SENSORY MOTOR INTEGRATION AND HEARING

BETTY PETERSEN

BECAUSE IT IS the only institution of its kind in the county offering audiological and educational services, San Diego Speech and Hearing Center has seen hundreds of hearing-impaired children on a nonselective basis. For the past eight years, all children, regardless of etiology or complaint, have received similar diagnostic testing, audiological services and education. I believe we have an excellent record for differential diagnosis and amplification procedures. While the educative procedures are not as complete as desired, we have helped many children, using auditory-oral methods, to attain speech and language.

Since we use the same procedures and methods for all children, we are concerned with the unsuccessful child. You recognize him . . . he may imitate and repeat but not remember. He may repeat backwards; 'shif' for fish, 'markbook' for bookmark. His auditory skills may be limited to very gross discrimination. He may be hyperkinetic, passive, irritable, impulsive, frustrated, distractible, tunes in and out, inattentive; he doesn't pay attention. The questions of how he differs in his response to the auditory-oral program could not be immediately answered by differences in hearing loss, amplification, education or parent involvement. Rather than believe it is the auditory-oral method that fails, we have tried to look for other causes of failure.

A referral of a mildly cerebral palsied child to a sensory motor integration program at Children's Hospital opened up new avenues of investigation. Margaret was referred for exercises for her feet and other motor coordination problems. In less than six months, her verbal skills and auditory abilities improved. Measured by the ITPA, at 1 year, she averaged six months more than the expected gain. What happened to Margaret? After an evaluation of her individual needs, she received sensory input to enhance vestibular, tactile and kinesthetic integration.

This basic type of integration is felt to enhance visual and auditory functions. A treatment program, which looks like games played with interesting equipment, is developed with the child's needs and parent-home involvement in mind. Treatment may last six months or longer, depending on progress and severity of problems. Chart comments by a hearing therapist usually show that change comes quickly during the initial weeks because hearing therapy is scheduled immediately following sensory-motor therapy. In most of the children referred, we note similar changes in verbal and auditory skills and other areas such as hyperactivity, irritability, tactile responses and motoric status.

We began to observe children closely in the auditory test situation to see if we could predict which children were most likely to succeed in an auditory-oral program and which would need, in addition, a sensory motor integration program.

Based on observations over a two-year period, we noted ten areas in

Table XVI-I

SCALE FOR DIFFERENTIAL DIAGNOSIS

BETTY PETERSEN

MARY KAWAR O.T.R.

1	2	3
passive	Activity level	hyperactive
unresponsive	Tactile response	tactilly defensive
right only	Ability to cross midline	left only
delayed	Motoric status	impetuous
abnormal flexion	Postural movement and response	abnormal extension
does not look	Eye pursuit	visually distractible
hypotonic	Oral function	hypertonic
very flexible	Muscle tone	tight
passive	Emotional affect response	irritable
dry	Skin tone	very moist

which children could be rated on a continuum with the normal child being rated in the middle.

Based on this scale, a child too far to the right or too far to the left would be in need of a sensory motor integration program, whereas the child in the middle of the continuum would not.

Since the majority of children we see lose their hearing from illness or birth trauma or are born with hearing impairments due to fetal insult, the majority fall at the extremes. Some inherited deaf have appeared normal and thus fall in the center norm.

When hearing losses are due to insult and/or trauma, there also may be related neurophysiological or perceptual disorders. The disorders of integration may be visual, auditory, tactile, vestibular or kinesthetic. When I speak of vestibular, I refer to those receptors that tell us of our relationship to gravity, to the body's movement in space. When I speak of kinesthesia, I refer to those receptors that tell us of movement in our joints. Perception takes place at high levels of the brain, but there can be disorders of sensory integration, a lack of processing at lowel levels, at the brain stem, that interfere with learning.

Dr. Jean Ayers at USC has conducted a study to see if procedures of general sensory integration would facilitate learning. Those who received sensory motor training showed greater gains in auditory, language and reading skills than those who spent extra time in the classroom receiving special auditory and language training. Three concepts were used in Dr. Ayers' study:

1. Interdependence of the sensory systems. Maturation of auditory systems may be be dependent on maturation of other systems. The program may have helped *normalize* the other systems.
2. Development of higher intellectual functions will not occur readily unless the hemispheres are able to specialize in their functions and have good communication between them. Language is a bilateral function with both hemispheres of the brain working together.
3. Dependence of the cortex on the lower brain structure, especially the brain stem.
   Hypothesis—the better the lower levels work, the better cognitive levels function.

The sensory motor integration staff under Mary Kawar, Chief of Occupational Therapy, believe that the sensory motor integration program will enhance all the child's systems so that he can organize his world and act more purposefully in terms of his environment.

Here is an example of how this concept might work with an auditory problem: Jennifer was a seven-year-old who was having problems in school. She was referred by her otologist for a hearing aid fitting. She had a severely sloping reverse loss, 75 to 15 dB in the right ear. Her hearing was within normal limits in the left ear. There was no response to bone conduction, presumably because of a deficient tactile system. During the diagnostic therapy, it was noted that Jennifer was hyperactive and distractible. She was not a good lipreader. Her language and speech were fair. It was suggested that she have a sensory motor integration evaluation and a trial period of therapy. At the end of six months of therapy, she was retested with the following results. Both ears were within normal limits. There was an SRT of 15 dB. Considerable improvement was noted in her listening ability, behavior and school work. There was now response to bone conduction.

Mrs. Kawar believes that the brain is plastic and can be influenced by a sensory motor integration program. This concept of the capacity of the brain to learn new patterns is supported by research and by our own observations. They prefer to work with younger children of three or four years but have accepted older children into the program. One of these accepted recently was a twelve-year-old, severely hard of hearing child that we have worked with since he was discovered to have a loss at age five. John has a 60–75 dB loss in the right ear and a fairly flat 80–100 dB loss in the left ear. John's homelife is undesirable; his attendance at lessons is erratic. He has been difficult to fit with hearing aids, as there are tolerance problems. His understanding was poor. He scored *three years and six months* in auditory reception at age eleven. He was unable to repeat a sentence of more than four words without omissions or reversals. This year, after three months of sensory motor integration therapy, his social behavior is improved. He looks at you when he talks; he follows directions better. He can repeat eight words in a sentence. He now scores *nine years and four months* in auditory reception. He has gained three years in visual association and visual reception. The rest of the test has not been completed. He has three more months of sensory motor integration therapy.

Another child, Greg, was first seen at our center when he was two and one-half. He was so hyperactive that he was difficult to control. His responses to auditory testing were sporadic but always showed loss at 70 dB or more. We tried amplification. After one hour, he weared of sound and showed signs of blinking and extreme nervousness. He appeared to respond to background noises only. He was referred to the sensory motor integration program but dropped out in a few months. He was referred from one psychiatrist to another and to several speech clinics. His mother was also referred for psychiatric help. Language did not begin to develop until age five and that was largely due to his mother's efforts. At five and one-half years, he was seen again at our center for testing. A 35 to 65 dB loss was found in the left ear, and questionable response in two frequencies at 70 and 100 dB were noted in the right. We worked with the Hear Training Unit as our diagnostic tool and found that Greg *heard* better with his left hand. That is, his motoric response to a sound stimulus was better when he used his left hand. He heard and repeated but could not respond, or if he did, there was a long delay. There was no discrimination at all in the right ear. A very mild gain instrument was fitted to the left ear, but it did not prevent him from tuning in and out or listening only to background sounds. After many sessions with the hearing aid, he continued to repeat correctly what was said but handed me the wrong item. Visually he was able to remember thirteen items but it took months of laborious training to get him to remember three or four items auditorially. He remembered phrases better than single words. He was very hyperactive and silly, difficult to manage. I.Q. testing showed only 73.

We referred him again to sensory motor integration therapy. They found him tactilly defensive, compensating visually. He had poor postural movements and hypermobility of the joints. Motor performance tests were below norm. He was right-handed. He could not cross the midline. He could not relax.

Their goals were to relax him, integrate the primitive postural reflexes, increase his adaptive responses and improve attention span. After six months of sensory motor integration training, many of the goals were achieved or were within reach. We retested with the ITPA. Language responses during the previous testing had been limited. Now he was using four-word sentences although the syntax was still deviant. Auditory memory showed an increase of one year. Verbal expression increased two years and his rating changed from significant deficiency to normal. He gained *two years ten months* on grammatic skills. On audiological retest, the left remained unchanged, but the right ear now showed a significant improvement of 20 to 40 dB in all frequencies. He was fitted with a second aid with only slightly more gain than the first. Discrimination was beginning to develop in the right ear. Behavior had improved. He was only silly if he felt he could not perform adequately. He continued to do well in a learning disabilities class.

I would like to summarize my own concepts of what happened to these children:

The auditory system is the most sophisticated tactile system. It functions better when the underlying tactile systems function well.

Auditory skills, language skills and reading skills are bilateral functions of the hemispheres of the brain. When each hemisphere is performing its job in synchronization with the other, language develops more readily.

The brain can inhibit stimuli and needs to in order to attend to the important and difficult cognitive skills. Many of our children like Greg are taking in too much unimportant material. Because they are not inhibiting the unnecessary, the brain is too busy to integrate and organize cognitive matters.

The vestibular system is influenced by the hearing aids. (We have always noted a change in balance when aids were fitted binaurally.) Apparently enhancing that system has a great influence on auditory skills.

We feel this program has made significant changes in all the children involved, perhaps the primary area being cooperation. In some cases, sensory motor integration therapy has been indicated before hearing education can even begin. It has helped the overactive to inhibit their behavior. It has enhanced the inactive. Balance and muscle tone has improved. Bilateral functioning has improved. Oral function has improved. All the children have been noted to be happier and more alert and in many cases functional vocabulary has increased.

There are many areas for research, many hypotheses to prove, more concepts to develop. We feel very fortunate to have such a capable and innovative staff to work with us.

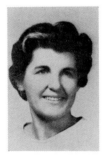

BETTY PETERSEN, A.B.

1942   A.B., San Diego State College, General Elementary Credential, Life
1948   Kindergarten–Primary requirements completed for Credential
1952   Guidance and Counseling, 9 units
1952   Supervision of student teachers
1953   Special Secondary Speech Correction Credential
1954   Lip Reading and Hard-of-Hearing, requirements completed for Credential
1954   Advanced Workshop for Deaf and Hard of Hearing, San Francisco State College, Basic Curriculum for Deaf and Hard of Hearing
1955   Audiology, requirements for Certificate completed, San Diego State College
1960   Neurologically Handicapped Children (Frostig Clinic) UCLA Course
1942–1946   1st grade, San Diego City Schools
1947–1948   Substituting, all grades, San Diego City Schools
1948–1954   Kindergarten, San Diego City Schools
1954–1955   Ungraded Oral Deaf, La Mesa-Spring Valley School District
1955–1963   HEAR Foundation, San Diego, California
1963–   Supervisor, Hearing Education Department, San Diego Speech and Hearing Center

Chapter XVII

AN ACOUPEDIC PROGRAM

Doreen Pollack

A COUPEDICS IS A program of educational audiology which is designed to meet the needs of children whose hearing losses are detected at an early age. It was so named by the late Dr. Henk Huizing of The Netherlands to differentiate it from traditional preschools for the deaf. This kind of program was only feasible after 1940 when personnel and equipment became available to test infant hearing and when powerful hearing aids were made which could be worn by infants.

An acoupedic program came into being to meet the challenge of progress in other areas. As the years went by, one idea led to another, and basic principles became crystallized.

The primary goal of an acoupedic program is to help children with residual hearing reach their true potential and stay, if possible, in the mainstream of our culture. It is necessary to work hard and consistently to reach that goal, and I might add, it is not possible to succeed without real commitment.

What are the main objectives of an acoupedic program? The *first* has to be the creation of the right learning environment. After many years in different settings, I discarded the idea of grouping young children with similar impairments and now advocate individualized training for many reasons:

a) An infant normally learns his communication in a process of unconscious identification with a mother figure. We have to develop the kind of close, warm, interpersonal relationships that foster oral communication. One has to teach infants with love.

b) The teacher and family can work together to create the best possible learning environment within each child's home. It has to be a family project.

c) The teacher can begin at the child's developmental level and build upon each child's abilities. In a one to one relationship, early diagnosis becomes possible of those other problems which tend to be overlooked in a group situation.

d) The young child's models for communication should be normal hearing, speaking and behaving. In a special preschool group, all the children have the same communication and behavioral problems. I have come to feel that there is little to be gained by that and a lot to lose if our goal is normal communication.

The second major objective is the development of an auditory function. By turning residual hearing into usable hearing, we integrate hearing into the total personality of a so-called deaf child. Although the importance of utilizing residual hearing has been recognized for centuries, the idea that hearing can be a major avenue for communication for the deaf is still so revolutionary that a recent report by Dr. Northern *et al.*, states that the failure of personal, auditory amplification programs is unfortunately common in schools for the deaf, and there is a vast number of older deaf students who could benefit from a personal hearing aid but do not have one. In one school, only 31 percent of the hearing aids were found to be in working order.

Ongoing audiologic assessment is essential to a successful acoupedic approach, but we have learned over the years not to place too much emphasis upon audiometric information. One cannot predict what a child will do,

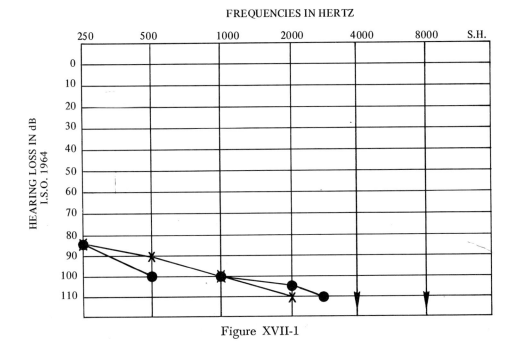

Figure XVII-1

* Northern, McChord, Fischer, and Evans: Hearing services in residential schools for the deaf. *Maico Audiological Library Services.* Vol. XI, Report Four.

in his brain, with the auditory signals which we can only measure at the level of the peripheral mechanism.

Here is the audiogram of a youngster who has been able to succeed

FREQUENCIES IN HERTZ

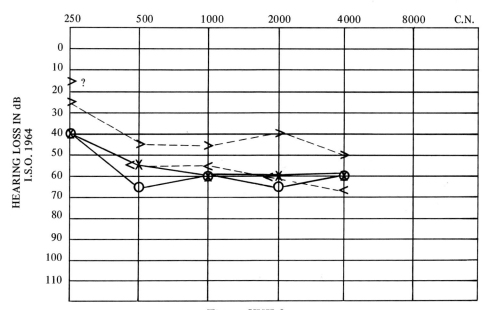

Figure XVII-2

FREQUENCIES IN HERTZ

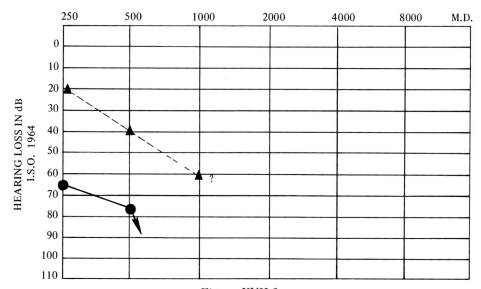

Figure XVII-3

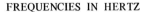

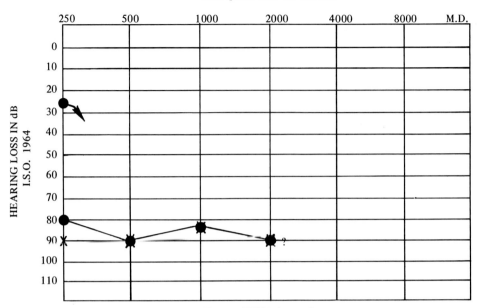

Figure XVII-4

without special education, has learned a foreign language and speaks so well that she has had a leading part in children's theatre. In contrast, here is the audiogram of a little girl who is only hard of hearing; however, she has had many learning problems and needs special education. (Figure XVII-2).

Early audiograms may change, not only because it is often difficult to obtain a reliable audiogram of an infant, but because of frequent conductive components which a preschooler eventually outgrows. (Figure XVII-3).

This child came to us with this audiogram obtained at a well known Medical Center. After myringotomies, her hearing acuity looked like this: (*See* Figures XVII-4 and XVII-5).

The first audiogram of this boy showed hearing only in one ear. We went ahead and fitted him binaurally, which was fortunate because at age seven, his audiogram looked like this. (*See* Figure XVII-6).

Having fitted hearing aids, we do not give sessions of auditory training nor divert the child's attention toward lipreading. For us, listening must be a continuous activity, part of everything we do. Many of our children wear their aids at night, too.

The auditory techniques we use are appropriate to the sequential stages involved in the development of an auditory function for a normal hearing infant in the first year of life.

FREQUENCIES IN HERTZ

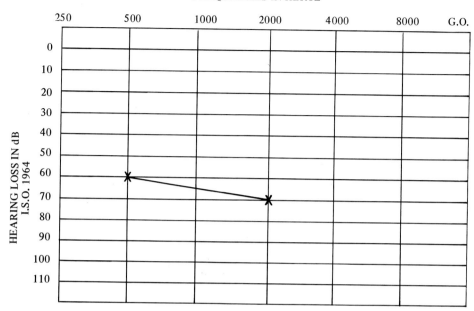

SPEECH AWARENESS: 75 dB.

Figure XVII-5

FREQUENCIES IN HERTZ

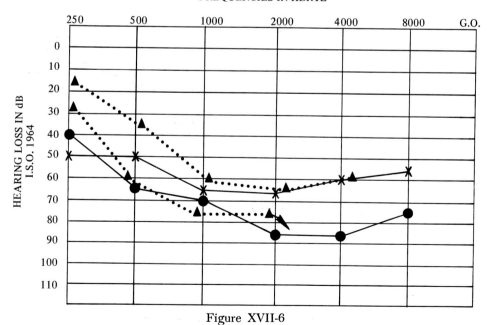

Figure XVII-6

The first step is *AWARENESS:* The infant must be made aware that sound is on, off, loud, quiet, rhythmic, noisy, male, female and so on. We clap our hands to our ears and say: "What's that? I hear that." Then we show him where the sound is coming from.

The next step is *ATTENTION* or learning to listen. A recent presentation at the ASHA Convention* showed that the pattern of evoked responses when the brain is just stimulated by sound is different from the pattern when the person is actively attending to the sound. We teach the child to attend to sound and respond to sound. Here begins also inhibition of response and separation of signal from the background noise. If we see a response at close range, we move the sound further and further away, and we move around the room and even outside the room. If the child does not localize, we turn him in the right direction.

The next major step is *DISCRIMINATION.* Having learned that the world is full of sounds, the infant must now learn that each sound has its own meaning. Discrimination seems to take place within the brain only after hundreds of hours of input, even for the normal hearing child, and it may take two years for a profoundly deaf youngster. But once an infant can discriminate, he can learn to babble, sing, whisper and imitate his first words. He will also develop an auditory feedback mechanism and monitor his own speech and language.

The attainment of oral communication is our next objective. A natural voice quality, well articulated speech and natural language may be attained through an auditory approach. Two more basic auditory skills are important: one is auditory memory, which involves both short term and long term memory, and also memory span. The other is sequencing, the ability to remember the exact sequence of sounds in a word and words in a sentence. There is no easy way to attain this objective. It takes many years of hard work; however, a child who can listen and imitate is free to learn wherever he goes and whatever he does.

The last major objective is integration. Preparing a child for the mainstream is not a denial of his hearing problem, but rather represents a viewpoint that the problem is only one part of a child: a handicap which may be overcome so that the hearing-impaired person is not restricted to a subculture unless he wishes to be. It gives him a choice.

Educational integration begins when we place the preschooler in a nursery school for normal hearing youngsters. As the fifth birthday approaches, we begin to prepare for kindergarten with an emphasis upon auditory skills which involve memorization, phonics, rhyming, questions and answers and so on. The i/t/a method of teaching reading has been a logical one for us to use since it is based upon sounding out words written in a phonetic alphabet. Once a child enters school, we continue to provide

---

* ASHA Convention, Robert Galambas, San Francisco, November,

support as necessary. One has to be careful to continue auditory training since a great deal of emphasis is placed upon visual skills in formal education.

Neither is integration unrealistic. Nine out of twelve children in the acoupedic program headed by Dr. Stewart in the early 1960's are still successful in their neighborhood schools and 22 out of 29 from the Porter Hospital Program. As you can see in the following table, the degree of hearing loss is not the criterion for successful integration. I must also emphasize that we see the children for only two or three sessions per week.

TABLE XVII-I

PORTER HOSPITAL
RESULTS OF ACOUPEDIC PROGRAM, 1972

Children who started as infants or preschoolers	Children who started in other programs	
	IN REGULAR SCHOOL	IN SPECIAL SCHOOL
MODERATE LOSS P/T Av. 55–70 dB.	8 + 2 (2)	
SEVERE LOSS P/T Av. 71–90 dB.	5 + 1 (6)	
PROFOUND LOSS P/T Av. 91–110 dB.	9 + 1 (6)	3 + 4

The challenge before us is to find ways to apply the successful techniques in a small program to the thousands of children in large school systems.

We have come to see clearly that there are three major factors for the success of an oral auditory approach: The most important factor concerns the parents and their goals. They have to want their child to talk and be willing to work hard for many years. They must also be able to establish an emotionally healthy parent-child relationship.

In support of the family, we offer the usual home visits, parent meetings and so on. In addition, we have two wonderful groups of volunteers to inspire parents and help them in many ways: the LISTEN FOUNDATION which was organized by parents in the program and the ECHO group which was formed by teenagers and young adults who had themselves received training in an acoupedic program. Representatives of these two groups are present at this Conference to share their ideas with you. ECHO, by the way, stands for Enthusiasm and Concern for Helping Others.

A second factor concerns the teacher: her goals, her commitment and her knowledge of young children. Many teachers, I am sorry to say, give up much too soon.

The third factor, of course, involves the child and what he brings into the program. We find we have two groups of children: one group consists of children who have a peripheral hearing loss but are otherwise intact, and the other consists of children whose hearing loss is secondary to central nervous system dysfunction and is part of a syndrome of learning disability. Since our program is in a hospital speech and hearing clinic, and we must accept all patients who are referred to us by physicians, it is possible we see more than our fair share of children with multiple handicaps, but there is at least one in every classroom. Mrs. Ernst, the educational audiologist on my staff, will now present an analysis of 23 children whose birthdates fell between 1964 and 1965.

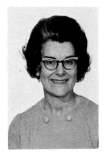

DOREEN POLLACK, B.A., L.C.S.T.

Doreen Pollack was educated in England and spent her early teaching years there. She holds a Diplomat Degree from London University. She came to the United States in 1948. She has worked in schools, universities, hospitals and other private agencies on both sides of the Atlantic. She has published numerous articles on speech pathology and audiology and is the author of a book: *Educational Audiology for the Limited Hearing Infant.* Mrs. Pollack is the Director of Speech and Hearing Services at Porter Memorial Hospital, Denver, Colorado, and also the wife of an engineer and mother of three children.

REPORT OF THE PORTER HOSPITAL STUDY OF HEARING-IMPAIRED CHILDREN BORN DURING 1964–65, INCLUDING THIRTEEN ACOUPEDICALLY TRAINED CHILDREN

MARIAN ERNST

THIS PAPER is a report of a recent study undertaken at Porter Memorial Hospital, Denver, Colorado. The purpose of this study was to illustrate how an auditory approach may be beneficial to all children regardless of the etiology of the hearing impairment or the severity of the hearing impairment itself.

The subjects of this study were twenty-three children who were born during the eighteen-month period between April 15, 1964, and November 15, 1965. The study is nonselective in that each child had only to be referred to the Porter Hospital Speech and Hearing Clinic because of hearing loss and participate in that hospital's therapy program.

The specific period of time for the study was chosen because of the large number of rubella children born during 1964-65 and because it has been suggested in the literature that many children in this group may also have other handicaps, including learning handicaps (Lehman and Simmons, 1972), in addition to their hearing impairments.

The subjects are listed in Table XVII-II by alphabetical code letters, the letters of the alphabet corresponding to the age of the child. Ages on January 1, 1973, ranged from seven years one month to eight years eight months. Degree of hearing loss is based upon the most recent audiological tests available for each child.

The average decibel loss for this group is 71 dB in the child's best ear, and the range of hearing loss is from 55 dB to 100 dB. Two of the multiply-handicapped children were later found to have hearing within the normal range. Etiology for the group is predominately rubella, with sixteen children identified as probable rubella babies. Prematurity was a factor for two children; hereditary deafness was present in four cases including one of Wardenburg's. In one case, Kanamycin was used, while the cause of hearing loss has never been identified for three children. Four children had obvious multiple handicaps. Hearing loss appeared to be the only symptom in the remaining nineteen cases.

Table XVII-II
Non-Selectivity of Cases[*]

CHILD	C.A. 1-1-73		Best Ear P.T. Ave.	Etiology	Initial Diagnosis
A	8 yr	8 mo	57 dB	Premature, Kanamycin	Deafness
B	8	8	80 dB	Rubella, Hereditary	Deafness
C	8	6	55 dB	Hereditary	Hard-of-Hearing
D	8	4	75 dB	Rubella-Premature	Deafness
E	8	3	100 dB	Rubella	Deafness
F	8	0	72 dB	Rubella	Deafness
G	8	0	82 dB	Rubella	Deafness
H	8	0	Within normal limits	Rubella	Multiply-handicapped, Deaf, Blind, Retardation
I	7	11	85 dB	Rubella	Deafness
J	7	11	93 dB	Rubella	Multiply-handicapped, Deaf, Autistic, Blind—one eye
K	7	11	57 dB	Rubella	Deafness
L	7	10	Within normal limits	Rubella	Multiply-handicapped, Retardation, Profound hearing loss
M	7	9	83 dB	Probably Rubella	Deafness
N	7	8	90 dB	Unknown	Deafness
O	7	8	75 dB	Rubella	Deaf–Blind
P	7	6	100 dB	Unknown	Deafness
Q	7	6	98 dB	Unknown	Deafness
R	7	3	95 dB	Rubella	Deafness
S	7	2	85 dB	Rubella	Deafness
T	7	2	95 dB	Rubella, Near drowning	Deafness
U	7	1	61 dB	Rubella	Deafness
V	7	1	70 dB	Hereditary	Deafness
W	7	1	95 dB	Wardenburg's Syndrome (Hereditary)	Deafness

[*]*Early-to-Read i/t/a Program.* New York, Initial Teaching Alphabet Publications, 1966.
Children are given Identification Letters which coincide with their chronological ages. The oldest child is identified as A, the youngest as W.

Pure-tone averages for the child's best ear are given **here** show the child's response to sound *after* training. Initial pure-tone and free-field tests often indicated much more profound hearing losses especially for the multiply-handicapped. Not reflected here is the

Of the total number, thirteen children entered the Acoupedic Program. The acoupedic group is characterized by early identification of hearing loss, early fitting of binaural hearing aids and early entrance into the training method which has been described as the Acoupedic Approach (Pollack, 1970). Table XVII-III shows the children who entered this program. The average hearing loss for this group was 79 dB for the best ear, although the loss of hearing ranged from 57 dB to 100 dB. Hearing loss was detected as early as the day of birth for one infant through the Neonatal Screening Program (Downs and Sterritt, 1967) and as late as two years one month for another. Detection of hearing loss for the group averaged one year and two-and-one-half months. Hearing aids, in most cases binaural, were fitted on an average of four-and-one-half months after detection, and training began approximately three months later. The average age for beginning auditory experience was twenty months, although the youngest had begun by eight months, and the oldest did not enter until two years seven months of age. Using hearing age as a measure of these children's auditory experience, it can be seen that they have experienced from four years seven months to seven years two months of auditory environment by January 1973. Their actual chronological ages average less than two years greater than their hearing age.

Children who have left the program at Porter Hospital prior to January 1, 1973, are listed in Table XVII-IV. Three children left the Denver area, three are presently in the Regional Deaf-Blind Program and one child left to enter a special education classroom for the hearing-impaired. One other child left the program because of lack of transportation. Because some follow-up data is available for Children A, C and D, these children will be included in later portions of the study. Children H, L, O, S and W will be deleted from further study.

When children are identified as suffering from hearing loss, fitted with hearing aids and provided with appropriate training early in life, it is felt that the outlook for their eventual remediation will be far more favorable than it would have been had these procedures not been followed; however, the presence of secondary factors influencing the child's development must always be considered. Of the thirteen children who entered the Acoupedic Program, five of them eventually developed secondary problems which marked them as deviating significantly from the pattern of development expected of children who are stimulated to learn auditorily.

Of the five children shown in Table XVII-V, four of them developed problems which significantly inhibited their learning. Three of these children remained highly echolalic and failed to move on the symbolic level of language. Child B, for example, learned a small vocabulary of a dozen nouns through extensive repetition and a few cliches which she used situ-

Table XVII-III

THE ACOUPEDIC GROUP:

*Early Identification and Training—Children who Entered by Three-and-a-Half Years of Age**

CHILD	BEST EAR P.T. AVE.	AGE PROBLEM WAS IDENTIFIED	AGE OF FITTING HEARING AID	AUDITORY STIMULATION BEGAN	PRESENT HEARING* AGE	PRESENT CHRONOLOGICAL AGE
		1 yr 3 mo	2 yr 3 mo	2 yr 5 mo	6 yr 3 mo	8 yr 8 mo
A	57 dB	1 – 0	1 – 6	1 – 7	7 – 1	8 – 8
B	80 dB	1 – 3	1 – 4	2 – 8	5 – 8	8 – 4
D	75 dB	1 – 5	1 – 6	2 – 3	6 – 0	8 – 3
E	100 dB	1 – 0	1 – 1	1 – 1	6 – 11	8 – 0
F	72 dB	1 – 2	1 – 9	1 – 9	6 – 2	7 – 11
K	57 dB	2 – 1	2 – 3	2 – 4	5 – 5	7 – 9
M	83 dB	1 – 6	1 – 11	1 – 10	5 – 10	7 – 8
N	90 dB	Day of Birth	– 4	– 8	6 – 10	7 – 6
P	100 dB	1 – 10	2 – 6	2 – 7	4 – 7	7 – 2
S	85 dB	1 – 0	2 – 1	1 – 2	4 – 11	7 – 1
U	61 dB	1 – 2	1 – 5	1 – 5	5 – 8	7 – 1
V	70 dB	1 – 0	1 – 5	1 – 5	5 – 8	7 – 1
Ave. for this group	79 dB	1 – 2	1 – 7	1 – 10	5 – 11	7 – 9

*The date auditory stimulation began coincides with the child's entrance to the therapy program at Porter Hospital for all children except Child V, who, although stimulated auditorily, did not enter the program until three years, one month of age.

Table XVII-IV

CHILDREN WHO LEFT THE PROGRAM PRIOR TO JANUARY 1, 1973*

CHILD	ENTRANCE AT AGE	LEFT AT AGE	LENGTH OF TIME IN PROGRAM	ATTENDANCE	REASON FOR LEAVING AND PRESENT PROGRAM, IF KNOWN
A	2 yr 5 mo	6 yr 5 mo	4 yr	Good	Left Area
C	6 – 11	8 – 3	1 – 4	Poor	Lack of home support
D	2 – 3	5 – 10	3 – 7	Good	Entered special class, Hearing-impaired
H	1 – 4	5 – 10	4 – 6	Good	Entered Regional Deaf-Blind Program
L	1 – 7	5 – 11	4 – 4	Fair	Entered Regional Deaf-Blind Program
O	2 – 10	5 – 4	2 – 6	Good	Entered Regional Deaf-Blind Program
S	2 – 7	4 – 2	1 – 7	Good	Left area, present placement unknown
W	1 – 5	4 – 2	2 – 8	Good	Left area, last known placement, special class for deaf

* Children A, C and D will reappear in later portions of this study.

ationally, while Child U perseverated extensively in all language activities. Child P, on the other hand, learned some words by age three and then lost all her early vocabulary. Children B, D, P and U had extensive problems with memory and sequencing of both the auditory and visual pathways. In contrast, Child M moved rather rapidly through the receptive portion of the Acoupedic Program but failed to develop expressive language. Problems of oral-apraxia appeared to be inhibiting his development of verbal language. In every case the clinician teaching these children was aware of these problems by four years of age and referred them for further testing. Except to confirm the presence of these problems, specific recommendations were made only in the case of Occupational Therapy Evaluations. Motor difficulties, including problems of dominance, bilateral integration, poor body schema and poor motor planning, characterize this group. Intersensory integration deficit appears to be a factor for all of the children. It should be noted that four of the five children presented here are of rubella etiology, and the case history for the fifth child suggests the presence of genetic factors related to learning.

A differential treatment program for these children was devised in the clinic and by age five all of them were participating in this program. Table XVII-VI briefly describes the program for each child. McGinnis techniques for the training of aphasic children were primarily utilized (McGinnis, 1963; Monsees, 1972). In addition, the *i/t/a reading program* was also successfully incorporated in this teaching. The *i/t/a reading system* is also used in this clinic with many other children who have no secondary learning problems. The Occupational Therapy recommendations were followed only in the case of Child M, whose training in this area has been found to be highly beneficial.

The results of this treatment program are shown in Table XVII-VII. All of those children who remained in the treatment program to present have developed receptive language vocabularies as shown by the scores on the Peabody Picture Vocabulary Test. In addition, everyone in this same group uses speech as the main mode of communication. Only Child M was felt ready for regular class placement with normal children. Children B, P and U were placed in special classrooms which were felt to better meet their present needs. Teacher ratings of these children have been very favorable, and all of the teachers have expressed enthusism for the child's ability to function in their classrooms. When asked to rate the child against other children of a similar age whom the teacher has taught in that particular type of educational setting, all of the teachers rated the children as average or above.

Of the thirteen original children in the Acoupedic Program, five of them have remained in the clinic program and have developed no secondary

Table XVII-V

ACOUPEDIC CHILDREN IN WHOM A SECONDARY PROBLEM WAS IDENTIFIED*

CHILD	BEST EAR P.T. AVE.	AGE ACOUPEDIC TRAINING BEGUN	AGE WHEN SECONDARY PROBLEM WAS IDENTIFIED	DESCRIPTION OF THE NATURE OF THE SECONDARY PROBLEM
B	80 dB	1 yr 7 mo	3 yr 6 mo	Echolalic. Problems of memory and retention. Failure to move on to symbolic level of language. Oral sensory feedback and motor planning for speech poor. Poor sequencing ability. Perceptual-motor disorder with lack of bilateral integration. Dominance not established. Deficiency in tactile perception, poor motor planning. Kinesthesia and visual perception lagging. Perseveration present. Visual memory poor. Letter reversals present to date (after four years experience). Occupational therapy recommended. Etiology: Hereditary and rubella.
D	75 dB	2 yr 8 mo	3 yr 6 mo	Echolalic. Problems of memory and retention. Failure to integrate symbolic language. Both auditory and visual pathways involved. Sequencing and categorization ability affected. Dominance not established. Chronic enuresis. Ileostomy, December 1971. Etiology: Rubella, premature.
M	83 dB	2 yr 3 mo	4 yr	Apraxia. Family history of late walkers and talkers. Difficulties in motor planning and delayed neuro-muscular action. Little bilateral integration. Tactile defensiveness exhibited, unable to integrate tactile information. O.T. evaluation, "Dysfunction lies within intersensory integration mechanism." Etiology: Probably rubella.
P	100 dB	8 mo	3 yr	Lost early vocabulary. Extensive problems of memory and retention. Aphasic. Poor tongue control and poor motor planning for speech. Very poor temporal sequencing ability. Dominance not established. Distractible but no major perceptual-motor deficiency. Father history of agraphia. Etiology: Unknown.
U	61 dB	2 yr 2 mo	4 yr	Extensive perseveration. Echolalic. Difficulties in retention of symbolic language. Poor temporal sequencing ability. Dominance not established. Etiology: Rubella.

* Child A is also known to have had mild perceptual problems; however, no information is available on the extent of treatment of these problems beyond the fact that the child is known to have had some special help in conjunction with his school program in a regular classroom.

Table XVII-VI

DIFFERENTIAL TREATMENT PROGRAM FOR ACOUPEDICALLY-TRAINED CHILDREN
WITH SECONDARY PROBLEMS

CHILD	DIFFERENTIAL TREATMENT BEGAN	DIFFERENTIAL TREATMENT TERMINATED	DESCRIPTION OF TREATMENT PROGRAM
B	4 yr 7 mo	To present	Differential Program for Aphasic Children (McGinnis, Monsees) to present. i.t.a. reading. Bilateral writing. Montessori training.
D	4 – 10	After one year entered special class, hearing-impaired	Differential Program for Aphasic Children to June 1970. Bilateral writing.
M	5 – 1	To present	Training for Oral Apraxia to present. i.t.a. reading.
P	4 – 7	To present	Differential Program for Aphasic Children to present. i.t.a. reading. Bilateral writing. Montessori training.
U	5 – 1	To present	Differential Program for Aphasic Children to present. i.t.a. reading. Bilateral writing.

problems. This group then represents the model in terms of setting the expectation levels and eventual goals for acoupedically-trained children. Table XVII-VIII describes this group. The degree of hearing loss is not felt to be a factor in the eventual success of the child. The hearing losses for children in this group range from 57 dB to 100 dB in the best ear. Of significance is early detection, fitting and training. The children's hearing ages for several children correspond to their Peabody scores. Regular class placement is not only possible but highly advisable as will be seen later when teacher evaluations of these children are presented. In every case, home support has been good, although individual parents support the program and expand the child's experiences in different ways. Parent education may be a factor as it is for any child, but concern for the child and willingness to spend the time to help him grow is probably more significant.

The remaining seven children not yet reported in this study entered the clinic after five years of age. This group is presented in Table XVII-IX. These children offer a basis for comparison on several factors felt to be significant in an Acoupedic Program. As a group, their degree of hearing loss is comparable to the acoupedic group, as is the time for detection of the presence of that loss. Of significance is the lateness in fitting hearing aids and commencing auditory stimulation. As a group, first hearing aids were fitted a year and nine months later than the acoupedic group, and in two cases, fitting was not done until six years of age. Even if an aid was fitted, as in the case of Child I, auditory treatment was often delayed until very late. Emotional problems, which have been virtually non-existent for the acoupedic group, once the child settled down and began to listen, have been more prevalent and in some cases, the overriding factor in therapy. It has been interesting to observe these children. Child C's problem was obviously detected late. On the other hand, Children G and Q had had sufficient auditory experience so that they have become programmed with the acoupedic group, now of school age. In spite of their late start, Children I and J are learning to listen and develop some receptive vocabularies commensurate with their hearing ages. These two children, along with children R and T, are presently in special education classes and are the subject of Table XVII-X.

Had Child I begun in an auditory program, he quite possibly would be participating in a regular class setting today. He is bright, has no secondary problems other than emotional ones tied to his late start and he has good home support. However, his communication skills do not reflect the fact that his hearing loss was detected at nine months of age.

Upon entering the clinic Child J had no vocabulary, receptively or expressively, and no communication skills apart from pulling or pushing

Table XVII-VII
SUCCESS OF TREATMENT FOR SECONDARY PROBLEM*

CHILD	C.A.	PEABODY M.A.	MODE OF COMMUNI-CATION	EDUCATIONAL PLACEMENT OF CHILD	NO. IN CLASS**	TEACHER FEELS CHILD WILL BE SUCCESSFUL	Progress Rating:	PARENTS FEEL CHILD IS PROPERLY PLACED	COMMENTS
B	8 yr 8 mo	3 – 6	Speech	Special classroom for children with learning problems. Moved to special class, Aurally Handicapped-Total commmunication	3 – 6	Yes	3	No	Recently moved to district with Oral Program
D	8 – 4	—	Jargon, some speech	Special class, hearing-impaired	—	—	—	Yes	Concern for child's physical health overrides educational considerations.
M	7 – 9	4 – 6	Speech	Regular first grade classroom, individual instruction from teacher-aide 20 minutes a day.	29	Yes	3 – 4	Yes	Very rapid progress last six months.
P	7 – 6	3 – 4	Speech, vocal emphasis	Special Class, Multiply Handicapped, not Hearing-Impaired	1 – 9	Yes	4 – 5	Yes	Very rapid progress last three months. At age in all academics except reading.
U	7 – 1	3 – 2	Speech	Special Class, Oral Program for Hearing-Impaired Normal kindergarten one hour a day.	4 – 23	Yes	4	Yes	Teacher comment: "Doing beautifully."

* All rating scales used in this study are ranked on a one-to-five scale as follows:
1. Lowest 10%   3. Average   5. Top 10%
2. Below average 4. Above average for the group
Information on Child D which was teacher supplied is unavailable.
** In the column "No. in Class," the first number for Children B and P indicates the number of children in the child's instructional group. The second number indicates the number in the group for other group activities. The first number for Child U indicates the number in her special class; the second, the number she participates with in her kindergarten class.

Table XVII-VIII
ACOUPEDIC GROUP–NO SECONDARY PROBLEMS*

CHILD	BEST EAR P.T. AVE.	HEARING AGE	PEABODY M.A.	C.A.	CLASS PLACEMENT REGULAR SCHOOL	FAMILY SUPPORT	PARENT EDUCATION	
							Mother	Father
E	100 dB	6 yr	4 yr 6 mo	8 yr 3 mo	2nd	Good stable home	Business college, one year	High School
F	72 dB	6 – 11	7 – 6	8 – 0	2nd Reading 3rd	Excellent home support	College; Graduate School	L.L.B. and M.A.
K	57 dB	6 – 2	5 – 8	7 – 11	1st	Home unstable; Mother supportive	Business college, one year	M.A.
N	90 dB	5 – 10	5 – 6	7 – 8	1st	Excellent; father takes active role	College, freshman yr.	College, freshman year
V	70 dB	5 – 8	5 – 5	7 – 1	1st	Excellent support; mother oral-deaf	M.A.	College, junior year
Average for the group	78 dB	6 – 1	5 – 8	7 – 9				

* Peabody Mental Age Scores for Children E and F do not correspond to their present chronological ages. These scores are, however, the most recently available.

Table XVII-IX

CHILDREN WHO ENTERED PORTER PROGRAM AFTER FIVE YEARS OF AGE°

CHILD	ENTERED PORTER AT AGE	BEST EAR P.T. AVE.	HEARING LOSS IDENTIFIED AT AGE	FITTED WITH AID AT AGE	PRIOR PROGRAMS
C	6 yr 4 mo	55 dB	5 yr	6 yr 6 mo	No
G	6 — 6	82 dB	2 — 6	2 — 9	Yes
I	5 — 3	85 dB	— 9	2 — 9	Yes(3)
J	5 — 8	93 dB	3 — 0	6 — 0	Yes
Q	5 — 2	98 dB	— 11	1 — 5	Yes
R	7 — 0	95 dB	3 wk.	— 11	Yes
T	5 — 6	95 dB	1 — 6	3 — 4	Yes
AVE.	5 — 11	86 dB	1 — 11	3 — 5	

°"Hearing Age" used here refers to the commencement of the use of meaningful auditory stimulation in the child's daily life, not the date when the child was fitted with an aid. "Hearing Age" is not a meaningful measure for Child C who heard well enough before his hearing loss was detected to have developed speech. Child C is not included in the group averages for Hearing Age, M.A. or C.A.

others about. In the two years since she has had her own hearing aids, she has learned to echo speech sounds and words clearly and intelligibly. She has a limited expressive vocabulary, and she will now tell you to "cut," "come," "down" and "cookie." More normal inflection patterns are becoming apparent all the time. Emotional problems, however, make her very difficult to program educationally. She cannot be taught in a group, and that fact places great restrictions not only upon her social and emotional development but communication as well.

Child R is doing very well where she is presently placed, but whenever a child is placed *specially*, the problems of normalization become greater as the child grows older. The question might be asked, "Are the goals appropriate? When is the best time to alter the goals set for a child and begin to program upwards?"

Child T, on the other hand, requires much special teaching and will need special class placement for some time.

Table XVII-XI describes ten of the original children in this study who now attend regular classes. Although the average hearing loss for this

METHOD OF TREATMENT	AUDITORY TREATMENT BEGAN	HEARING AGE	PEABODY M.A.	C.A.	OTHER PROBLEMS
----	6 yr 6 mo	----	5 – 11	8 – 6	Home unstable; 2 younger brothers also have hearing losses
Lipreading; Auditory	2 – 9	5 – 3	5 – 9	8 – 0	None
Lipreading	5 – 3	2 – 8	2 – 11	7 – 11	Emotional
Autistic; Non-directive	5 – 8	2 – 3	2 – 10	7 – 11	Emotionally disturbed Blind—one eye
Listening; Reading	2 – 6	5 – 0	5 – 1	7 – 6	None
Lipreading; Auditory	1 – 0	6 – 3	3 – 5	7 – 3	None
Lipreading; Listening	3 – 4	3 – 10	2 – 2	7 – 2	No mother; erratic attendance and behavior problems until recently
	3 – 11	4 – 2	3 – 6	7 – 7	

group is 77 dB, the degree of hearing loss ranged from 55 dB to 100 dB in the child's best ear. Hearing ages average five years, ten months for the group as a whole. Peabody scores are no longer given as mental ages, but as percentiles so that this group may now be compared with their own chronological age group. At this time, the children tend to be in the lowest ten percent for their own age group, with an average of 5 percent for the group as a whole with one notable exception.

The children attend seven different public schools in four different suburban Denver school districts. Two attend parochial schools, and one child attends a private school. Seven of the children are placed one grade below their age in keeping with the general policy that most hearing-impaired children will do better if they wait until seven years of age before entering first grade. Three children are, however, at age for their grade placement. The classes which these children attend are of a wide variety and include classrooms described as Self-contained, Team-teaching and Open-living which means that individual children vary in the number of social contacts they have within their school day. One class was described as a *low* class, another as a *high* class and one class is a first and second grade combination. Of the original acoupedic group of thirteen children, seven are now attending regular school. All of the parents have expressed satisfaction with their child's placement, although one parent felt that a more sympathetic teacher would improve her child's school situation.

Table XVII-X

SPECIAL EDUCATIONAL PLACEMENT FOR FOUR LATE-ENTERING CHILDREN NOT IN REGULAR SCHOOL

CHILD	SCHOOL PLACEMENT	MODE OF COMMUNICATION	TEACHER RATINGS						TEACHER COMMENT
			AGAINST HIS POTENTIAL			COMPARED WITH OTHERS			
			Acad.	S-E	Comm.	Acad.	S-E	Comm.	
I	Special Language Class—Not Hearing-Impaired	Jargon—Some Speech	4	3	2	4	3	2	Verbal skills improving but needs much encouragement.
J	Special Class Multiply-Handicapped Not Hearing-Impaired	Drawing, Isolated Words, Emotional Response, Screaming	1–5	3	2	3–4	1	1	Very difficult to rate. Far from where she was but a long way to go. Growing receptively. Socially not developing. Teacher considers child's principal problem to be emotional.
R	Oral Special Class, Hearing-Impaired	Speech	5	4	5	5	4	5	Top of her class of eight.
T	Special Oral Class Hearing-Impaired	Jargon, gestures, very little intelligible speech	2	4	1–2	3	4	2	Has good conceptual background and strong desire.

Table XVII-XI

CHILDREN WHO PRESENTLY ATTEND REGULAR CLASSES WITH NORMAL-HEARING CHILDREN*

CHILD	BEST EAR P.T. AVE.	HEARING AGE	PEABODY %	GRADE	TYPE OF CLASS	IN ACOUPEDIC GROUP	PARENT FEELS CHILD IS PROPERLY PLACED
A	57 dB	6 yr. 3 mo.	----	2nd	Regular school	Yes	Yes
C	55 dB	-------	6%	2nd	Low class	No	-------
E	100 dB	6 – 0	2%	2nd	Self-contained	Yes	Yes
F	72 dB	6 – 11	85%	2nd	Flexible; reads with third grade	Yes	Yes
G	82 dB	5 – 3	8%	1st	Self-contained	No	Yes
K	75 dB	6 – 2	4%	1st	Team-teaching	Yes	Yes
M	83 dB	5 – 5	1%	1st	High class	Yes	Yes
N	90 dB	5 – 10	4%	1st	Combination first and second	Yes	Yes
O	98 dB	5 – 0	3%	1st	Self-contained	No	Yes
V	75 dB	5 – 8	12%	1st	Open living	Yes	Yes
Ave. for this group	77 dB	5 – 10	5%				

* Although Children G and Q were not in the original acoupedic group, earlier training and stress on auditory skills with home support made regular class placement possible.

Feedback from the teachers about how they feel these children are doing was felt to be essential to this study, and these results are given in Table XVII-XII.

Teachers were asked to rate the child on a one-to-five rating scale as to his academic performance, his social and emotional adjustment and his communication ability. Because of the problems of objectivity involved when a teacher is asked to rate a child she knows is working under a handicap, each teacher was asked to first rate the child in each of the three areas, taking his handicap into consideration and evaluating what she felt the child was able to put into the situation. Teachers were then asked to rate the child again, this time against his classmates. For both evaluations, the tendency was to rate the child in most areas as average or above for his class. Most teachers felt that these children as a group were putting a lot into the situation and tended to give higher ratings when they could consider the fact that the child did have to work under a handicap. Teacher comments were also favorable and reflected that the teachers found the experience of teaching a hearing-impaired child profitable to themselves and to the child's classmates as well.

In summary, this study attempted to evaluate twenty-three children who were born between April 15, 1964, and November 15, 1965, and who were referred because of hearing loss for therapy at Porter Hospital, Denver, Colorado.

Of this group, sixteen were classified as rubella in terms of etiology, four as hereditary, one used Kanamycin and in three cases etiology was unknown. Of the rubella group, four were multiply-handicapped, and four were later found to develop secondary handicaps. Eight children left the program, three of whom entered programs for deaf-blind children, with follow-up being unavailable for two others.

Thirteen of these children entered the Acoupedic Program, with hearing losses ranging from 57 dB to 100 dB. Three of the acoupedic group left the program, while five other children in this group developed a secondary handicap in addition to hearing loss. Seven of these children now attend regular classes with normal-hearing children.

Seven children entered the program after four years of age. Delayed auditory experience was felt to be a crucial factor in the eventual progress of this group.

Of the original twenty-three children, ten are now placed in regular schools. Teacher ratings tend to place the performance of these children as average or above when compared with their hearing classmates. Teacher comments reflected positive attitudes towards integrating these children educationally. Success in this program was determined by early detection, early amplification and early training. Degree of hearing loss was not

Table XVII-XII

TEACHER RATINGS OF HEARING-IMPAIRED CHILDREN IN REGULAR CLASSES WITH NORMAL-HEARING CHILDREN

CHILD	BEST EAR P.T. AVE.	Child Rated Against His Potential			Child Rated Against His Classmates			COMMENTS
		ACAD.	SOC-EMOT.	COMM.	ACAD.	SOC-EMOT.	COMM.	
C	55 dB	2	3	2–3	3	3	2–3	Teacher could be more sympathetic; late identification, child needs much support.
E	100 dB	4	5	4	3	5	3	"She misses out at times but really very normal. Very popular."
F	72 dB	4–5	3	3	4–5	3	4	"Very superior. Tops in reading and language. May choose to read a book rather than participate in class discussion."
G	83 dB	3	4	3	3	4	2–3	"Tends to pull out when she does not wish to participate. Generally doing quite well."
K	57 dB	4	2	4	3	3	2	"His vocabulary limits his comprehension at times, but no question that child will be successful."
M	83 dB	4	4	3–4	3	4	4	"Participates and contributes as much as any child. Other children express much concern and empathy. Will be on year-round school. Not ready for team-teaching."
N	90 dB	5	5	3	4	5	2	"Competition for communication is very high in this class. Child has to work hard to get his chance. Very out-going, always tries."
Q	98 dB	3	3	3	3	3	4	"Has some problems socially and emotionally. Tends to like things rather rigid. Hears but does not really listen to others. Very tenacious. Will stay with things until he has them but feels he is somewhat too concerned about right and wrong."
V	75 dB	4–5	4	5	3–4	2	3	"Speaks right up. Can explain his feelings. Knows when he is not speaking clearly and works at it."

considered a significant factor in determining the child's eventual level of achievement.

REFERENCES

Early-to-Read i/t/a Program. New York, Initial Teaching Alphabet Publications, 1966.

Downs, M.P. and Sterritt, G.M.: A guide to newborn and infant screening. *Arch Otolaryng, 85:*210–213, 1967.

Lehman, Jean Utley and Simmons, M. Patricia: Comparison of rubella and non-rubella young deaf adults: Implications for learning. *Journal of Speech and Hearing and Hearing Research, 15:*734–742, 1972.

McGinnis, Mildred A.: *Aphasic Children: Identification and Education by the Association Method.* 1963.

Monsees, Edna K.: *Structured Language for Children with Special Language Learning Problems.* 1972.

Pollack, Doreen: *Educational Audiology for the Limited Hearing Infant.* 1970.

Chapter XVIII

LEARNING TO PROCESS AUDITORY INFORMATION

LEAHEA F. GRAMMATICO

HEARING IS THE fastest way to acquire information. The residual hearing of the hearing-impaired child can usually be developed to a functional level through consistent, continuous and appropriately selected amplification, coupled with a hierarchical arrangement of teaching learning experiences. Educational experiences that enable children to become contributing members of a highly technical society involve the development of listening skills, language and the expansion of language, speech and cognitive skills. The specific teaching strategies used to develop listening skills at Peninsula Oral School for the Deaf are cognitively based tasks, sequentially arranged and are based on Piaget's three major sequential steps of intellectual development and the Hilda Taba curriculum model. A child in the sensorimotor stage of development (birth to 18–24 months) obviously requires different teaching strategies than a child in the preconceptual phase of the concrete operations stage of development (18–24 months to 4 years). Contrary to the traditional approach of using noisemakers to develop the deaf child's residual hearing to a functional level, cognitive tasks, using only spoken voice, provide the content for developing listening skills. Noisemakers and speech are dissimilar phenomena. If listening is to become autonomous, it cannot be separated from the language, speech and cognitive facets of the curriculum.

Learning is hierarchical in nature and accumulates in the shape of an ascending spiral. Each stage of development is incorporated into the next higher stage. Unless specific teaching-learning experiences are devised that incorporate the stages of intellectual development with cognitive learning, high level abstractions (interdependence, change, comparisons (similarities and differences), cooperation, sequential order of events) cannot be acquired.

Each lesson given individually includes the following dimensions:

—Cognitive tasks involving problem solving, inference, classifying.

—Connected language

Single words do not provide enough information to develop listening skills, nor do they convey ideas.

—Intonational voiced patterns

Hearing-impaired children must learn to use their voices in a variety of ways to prevent acquiring *deaf speech*. Often the way something is said conveys as much meaning as what is said.

—Music

Songs in their entirety, i.e. "Happy Birthday," "Me and My Teddy Bear," "My Airplane Flys."

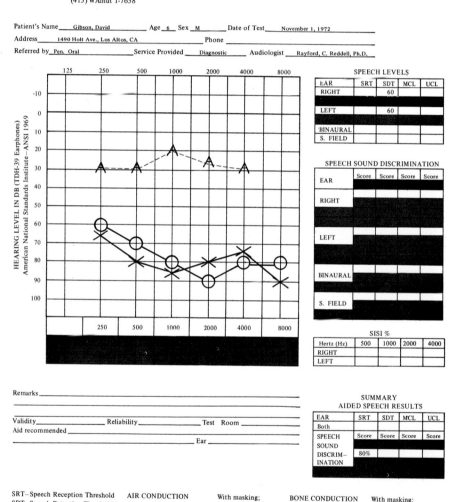

SAN FRANCISCO HEARING & SPEECH CENTER
2340 CLAY STREET, 6th FLOOR
SAN FRANCISCO, CALIFORNIA 94115
(415) WAlnut 1-7658

AUDIOLOGICAL TEST RESULTS

Patient's Name ___Gibson, David___ Age _6_ Sex _M_ Date of Test ___November 1, 1972___

Address ___1490 Holt Ave., Los Altos, CA___ Phone _____

Referred by ___Pen. Oral___ Service Provided ___Diagnostic___ Audiologist ___Rayford, C. Reddell, Ph.D.___

SPEECH LEVELS

EAR	SRT	SDT	MCL	UCL
RIGHT		60		
LEFT		60		
BINAURAL				
S. FIELD				

SPEECH SOUND DISCRIMINATION

EAR	Score	Score	Score	Score
RIGHT				
LEFT				
BINAURAL				
S. FIELD				

SISI %

Hertz (Hz)	500	1000	2000	4000
RIGHT				
LEFT				

Remarks _____

SUMMARY
AIDED SPEECH RESULTS

EAR	SRT	SDT	MCL	UCL
Both				

Validity _____ Reliability _____ Test Room _____

Aid recommended _____

_____ Ear _____

SPEECH SOUND DISCRIMINATION	Score	Score	Score	Score
	80%			

SRT—Speech Reception Threshold
SDT—Speech Detection Threshold
MCL—Most Comfortable Loudness
UCL—UnComfortable Loudness

AIR CONDUCTION
O Right ear (red)
X Left ear (blue)
S Sound field (unaided)
A Sound field (aided)

With masking;
Δ Right ear with masking in left
☐ Left ear with masking in right

BONE CONDUCTION
> Right ear (red)
< Left ear (blue)

With masking:
► Right ear with masking in left
◄ Left ear with masking in right

Table XVIII-I

—Speech.

Specific elements combined into finger play activities.

As listening skills develop, language and speech become clearer and more spontaneous involving the use of longer and more complex sentences. When the child has acquired some sophistication in listening, each dimension of the lesson gradually becomes increasingly complex. Listening de-

SAN FRANCISCO HEARING AND SPEECH CENTER
2340 CLAY STREET
SAN FRANCISCO, CALIFORNIA 94115
WAlnut 1-7658

REPORT OF AUDIOMETRIC EXAMINATION

Patient's Name ___Porter, Lisa_____ Age _5_ Sex _F_____ Date of Test ___12-29-70___

Address ___1148 Cedar, San Carlos 94070_____ Phone ___593-6433_____

Referred by___R. Perry, M.D._____ Service for which referred ___Diagnostic Audiologic Eval.___ Tested by ___R.C. Reddell, Ph.D___

Speech Reception thresholds: Right ear_____ Left ear_____70 dB_____ Sound field_____

Speech Sound Discrimination: Right ear_____ Left ear_____ Sound field_____

Estimate of validity:_____ Reliability: _____MCL: _____UCL _____

Aided Test Results: Speech Reception threshold:____15 dB_____ Discrimination_____ Ear:_____

Aid Recommended:_____ Ear: _____

Remarks:_____

_____

_____ Test   Rm. _____

(Arrows at top of audiogram indicate lateralization results of audiometric Weber test:→Right,←Left,←→ Center)

Table XVIII-II

velops from large pieces of information to smaller and smaller units—from sentences, to phrases, to words, to sounds.

The child's order of language output, however, is from sounds, to jargon, to words, to combining words; first two at a time, combining words with jargon, and then into longer and longer sentences that eventually increase in complexity.

SAN FRANCISCO HEARING AND SPEECH CENTER
2340 CLAY STREET
SAN FRANCISCO, CALIFORNIA 94115
WAlnut 1-7658

REPORT OF AUDIOMETRIC EXAMINATION

Patient's Name___CADEMATORI, Celeste_____ Age _5___ Sex _F___ Date of Test ___4-12-72_____

Address ___1550 Wakefield Terrace, Los Altos, CA_____ Phone ___967-0267_____

Referred by_Peninsula Oral School____ Service for which referred _Hearing aid_____Tested by ___Rayford C. Reddell, Ph.D
                                                          Consultation
Speech Reception thresholds: Right ear_75 dB_____ Left ear___75 dB_____ Sound field_____

Speech Sound Discrimination: Right ear_____ Left ear_____ Sound field_____

Estimate of validity: _____Reliability_____ MCL: _____ UCL _____

Aided Test Results: Speech Reception threshold: _30-35 dB_____Discrimination _____ Ear: _____

Aid Recommended: _____ Ear: _____

Remarks: _____

_____

_____ Test Rm. _____

(Arrows at top of audiogram indicate lateralization results of audiometric Weber test:→Right,←Left,↔Center)

Table XVIII-III

Child Response

The child who is learning to process information auditorily responds first to a spoken stimulus, such as his name, by dropping a ring onto a spindle. Secondly he enters the stage of imitation characterized by imitating syllables, ma, ma, ma, ma from da, da, da, da. He is also beginning to imitate intonational patterns but there is very little meaning attached to this voice play. In the third stage he is beginning to process information auditorily and visually. This stage is characterized by the use

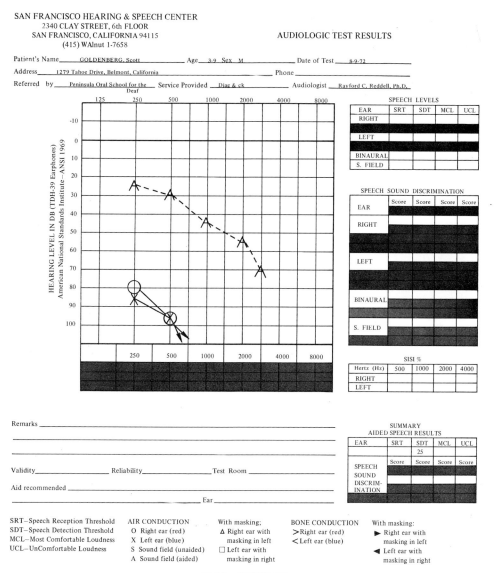

SAN FRANCISCO HEARING & SPEECH CENTER
2340 CLAY STREET, 6th FLOOR
SAN FRANCISCO, CALIFORNIA 94115   AUDIOLOGIC TEST RESULTS
(415) WAlnut 1-7658

Patient's Name ____GOLDENBERG, Scott____ Age__3-9 Sex_M____ Date of Test ___8-9-72___

Address____1279 Tahoe Drive, Belmont, California____ Phone ____

Referred by____Peninsula Oral School for the Deaf____ Service Provided __Diag & ck__ Audiologist __Rayford C. Reddell, Ph.D.__

SPEECH LEVELS

EAR	SRT	SDT	MCL	UCL
RIGHT				
LEFT				
BINAURAL				
S. FIELD				

SPEECH SOUND DISCRIMINATION

EAR	Score	Score	Score	Score
RIGHT				
LEFT				
BINAURAL				
S. FIELD				

SISI %

Hertz (Hz)	500	1000	2000	4000
RIGHT				
LEFT				

Remarks ____

SUMMARY
AIDED SPEECH RESULTS

EAR	SRT	SDT	MCL	UCL
		25		

	Score	Score	Score	Score
SPEECH SOUND DISCRIMINATION				

Validity____ Reliability____ Test Room ____

Aid recommended ____

____ Ear ____

SRT—Speech Reception Threshold
SDT—Speech Detection Threshold
MCL—Most Comfortable Loudness
UCL—UnComfortable Loudness

AIR CONDUCTION
O Right ear (red)
X Left ear (blue)
S Sound field (unaided)
A Sound field (aided)

With masking:
Δ Right ear with masking in left
□ Left ear with masking in right

BONE CONDUCTION
> Right ear (red)
< Left ear (blue)

With masking:
▶ Right ear with masking in left
◀ Left ear with masking in right

Table XVIII-IV

of what Gesell calls *expressive jargon* that becomes combinations of two words and then longer and longer sentences. He has learned that language has power and that he can manipulate and control his environment verbally. In the fourth stage he has acquired the sophisticated listening skills necessary to process information auditorily. A specific teaching strategy at this level might be changing the language of a familiar

SAN FRANCISCO HEARING & SPEECH CENTER
2340 CLAY STREET, 6th FLOOR
SAN FRANCISCO, CALIFORNIA 94115
(415) WAlnut 1-7658

AUDIOLOGICAL TEST RESULTS

Patient's Name Harbeson, Michael   Age 8-0   Sex M   Date of Test December 27, 1972

Address 27891 Lupine Rd., Los Altos Hills, CA 54002   Phone 541-4655

Referred by Penn. Oral   Service Provided DA & CK   Audiologist Rayford C. Reddell, Ph.D.

SPEECH LEVELS

EAR	SRT	SDT	MCL	UCL
RIGHT		90		
LEFT		90		
BINAURAL				
S. FIELD		40 dB	Aided	

SPEECH SOUND DISCRIMINATION

EAR	Score	Score	Score	Score
RIGHT				
LEFT				
BINAURAL				
S. FIELD				

SISI %

Hertz (Hz)	500	1000	2000	4000
RIGHT				
LEFT				

Remarks _____

SUMMARY
AIDED SPEECH RESULTS

EAR	SRT	SDT	MCL	UCL
SPEECH SOUND DISCRIMINATION	Score	Score	Score	Score

Validity _____ Reliability _____ Test Room _____

Aid recommended _____
_____ Ear _____

SRT—Speech Reception Threshold	AIR CONDUCTION	With masking;	BONE CONDUCTION	With masking:
SDT—Speech Detection Threshold	O Right ear (red)	Δ Right ear with	>Right ear (red)	▶ Right ear with
MCL—Most Comfortable Loudness	X Left ear (blue)	masking in left	< Left ear (blue)	masking in left
UCL—UnComfortable Loudness	S Sound field (unaided)	☐ Left ear with		◀ Left ear with
	A Sound field (aided)	masking in right		masking in right

Table XVIII-V

fairy tale. "Three prominent citizens of Greenwood Forest went for a walk early today. While they were gone their home was ransacked. Nothing of value appeared to be taken, but some food was eaten and a chair broken. The culprit was found asleep upstairs. You are urged to lock your house before leaving it." Did you know that this is the "Three Bears"?

Not every child will accomplish all four levels of behavior. Quantity and quality of residual hearing, age of onset of deafness, age of acquiring appropriate amplification, consistency in wearing his hearing aids or aid, quality and duration of educational experiences and the teacher's knowledge of amplifying systems will determine how functional each child's residual hearing will become.

Teacher Conduct

The development of sophisticated listening skills is dependent on diagnosis of needs, selection and organization of content, selection and organization of teaching learning experiences and evaluation of changing behavior. With the child who has just been diagnosed as deaf, or the young deaf child who has not yet acquired oral communicative skills, the content is in the form of labeling and relating concepts in words and meanings to the organizing facets of his environment—home, family, school, people, anatomy, clothes, food, transportation, toys, animals, illnesses, injuries, holidays, rules. In addition to organizing a total sequence of teaching-learning experiences that provides the means for acquiring knowledge, divergent and convergent thinking skills, attitudes, feelings and sensitivities and social and academic skills, the teacher must also acquire knowledge of the electroacoustic characteristics of amplifying systems.

Utilizing the Taba curriculum model, the plan devised for teachers for learning amplifications follows.

Basic Concepts
1) Change
2) Cooperation
3) Interdependence
4) Causality
5) Comparisons (similarities and differences)

Main Ideas
1) The development of listening skills is continuous, sequential and accumulative.
2) Only consistent, continuous and appropriately selected amplification will enable a child to develop his residual hearing to the greatest degree.
3) Appropriate amplification is not necessarily synonymous with power. Power is one facet of appropriate amplification as is selectivity.

4) An audiogram is limited in the information it provides. Expansion of the audiometric information is imperative for the development of sophisticated listening skills.
5) Children with identical audiometric measurements may require different amplifying systems to develop listening skills.
6) Even appropriately selected amplification is limited in value unless it is coupled with a hierarchical arrangement of teaching experiences.

Facts
1) Frequency response
2) Input
3) Output
4) Gain
5) Maximum power output

Otologists, audiologists, teachers, parents, engineers who design amplifying systems and makers of ear molds must work as a team if hearing-impaired children are to develop sophisticated listening skills. The otologist must be readily available to treat infections, remove cerumen and treat skin irritations that may result from certain ear molds. The audiologist is the specialist in hearing and hearing loss. He must interpret his clinical findings to the teacher, the person who is responsible for developing oral communicative skills. Parents must observe and assist teachers so that they can reinforce at home the oral communicative skills learned at school. The engineer cannot make changes in amplifying systems if he does not know that changes are needed. Not even the best amplifying system can provide quality amplification through a poor ear mold or collapsed tubing. Team effort is the key to providing appropriate amplification on a consistent and continuous basis if hearing-impaired children are to become contributing members of a changing technological society.

REFERENCES

Brown, Roger: *Social Psychology.* New York: The Free Press, 1965.
Davis, H. and Silverman, S.R.: *Hearing and Deafness,* revised ed. New York: Holt-Rinehart and Winston, Inc., 1970.
Hunt, J. McV.: *Intelligence and Experience.* New York: Ronald Press Co., 1961.
Krebs, Donald F.: *Ears Educational Amplification Response Study 1968.* Ears Monograph No. 1, 1968.
Phillips, John L.: *The Origins of Intellect—Piaget's Theory.* San Francisco: W.H. Freeman & Co., 1969.
Taba, Hilda: *Curriculum Development—Theory and Practice.* New York: Harcourt, Brace & World, Inc., 1962.
Taba, Hilda and Hills, James L.: *Teachers' Handbook for Elementary Social Studies.* Menlo Park: Addison-Wesley Publishing Co., 1967.

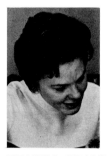

LEAHEA GRAMMATICO, M.A.

Mrs. Leahea F. Grammatico is director of the Peninsula Oral School for the Deaf. She is a graduate of Indiana State University, with a M.A. from San Francisco State University. Mrs. Grammatico believes that consistent and continuous and selected amplification coupled with consistent continuous teaching and learning experiences in the hands of creative teachers will produce outstanding oral deaf adults. Mrs. Grammatico was a high school science teacher, as well as a general elementary teacher, and has experience as a social worker and speech and hearing therapist. She holds three life credentials in the State of California in the areas of Education of the Deaf, Education of the Hard of Hearing and Elementary Education. She is also South-West Director A.O.E.H.I., Educational Consultant for the A.G. Bell Association, Consultant for Project NEED, University of Utah and Consultant, State Project EARS II.

Chapter XIX

THE INTEGRATED LINGUISTIC APPROACH TO THE SPEECH HABILITATION OF HEARING IMPAIRED CHILDREN

Djordje Kostić

DEAF CHILDREN, considered together, do not comprise a homogeneous, uniform population. In fact, the population which they do form does not consist of two simple, homogeneous subpopulations, one consisting of the totally deaf children and the other consisting of the hard of hearing or hearing-impaired children. The nature of this population is more complex than simple. This lack of universality applies to instructional methodology as well; there is no unique, universal method for teaching deaf children how to speak. Similarly, there is no single type of instrumentation which can be utilized for all hearing-impaired children. There is not just a single type of deafness, nor is there a single age of onset of deafness. There is not just one type of instrumentation for hearing-impaired children, nor is there a single, common basis for processing linguistic data. Instead, there are many of each of these, and none of them should be overestimated or underestimated.

In classifying hearing-impaired children, four dimensions need to be taken into account:

—age for onset of deafness
—damage to the auditory system, both quantitative and qualitative aspects
—ability to perceive and comprehend speech sounds and
—the time lag between the onset of deafness and the initiation of speech habilitation training.

In Yugoslavia, about 25 percent of the children attending special schools for the deaf require only linear amplification of sound for speech habilitation training. Another five percent are totally deaf and are unable to receive sound, regardless of the type of amplification. About 17 percent of the children in the special Yugoslav schools possess remnants of hearing which are just sufficient for coming into contact with sound but are insufficient for perception of speech sound quality. For about 28 percent of the children in the special schools, highly selective amplification of sound by means of an acoustic filter system is essential for speech habilitation training. The rest of the children fall between those who have sufficient remnants of hearing for speech habilitation using acoustic cues and those who are unable to utilize acoustic cues. They are the most complicated from the point of view of speech habilitation methodolgy and instrumentation, since they require the instrumentation appropriate for the totally deaf as well as the instrumentation appropriate for the hearing-impaired. In the Institute for Experimental Phonetics and Speech Pathology, Belgrade, an attempt is being made to construct words and sentences appropriate for such children by means of artificial speech sounds. These words and sentences are acoustically unlike those of everyday speech, but they possess acoustic elements sufficient for the organization of word and sentence meaning.

Deafness is customarily divided into two major types or classes, central and peripheral. Central deafness, being relatively rare, will not be dealt with further in this discussion. Peripheral deafness, which is the term used to characterize children with poor remnants of hearing, is of major concern when considering the speech habilitation of the hearing-impaired.

When dealing with the hearing-impaired child, it is customary to consider only the damaged auditory system, in particular the component parts of the ear, neglecting the basis for processing linguistic data within the child. Again, emphasizing the extent and intensity of damage to the ear, insufficient attention has been paid to the age for onset of deafness as a factor affecting the ability of the child to process linguistic data; furthermore, this factor is generally neglected as a classificatory dimension for hearing-impaired children.

Supposing that the fetus is able to react to external sound during the last few months before birth, as reported by Johannson, and supposing that it can sense or respond to the pulsation of the maternal heart, by the time that it is born, it will have had contact with an important phenomenon of speech, the rhythm which is closely related to the heart's pattern of pulsation. If a child is born without having had this prenatal physiological experience, then it will lack one of the crucial elements underlying the central nervous system's capability to process linguistic data, an element which may be presumed to be present in the normally-hearing, newborn child.

The hearing status of the child with no postnatal auditory experience is not the same as the hearing status of the child who loses the ability to perceive sound two months after birth. The latter child, within the first two months of life, is able to establish feedback control of its own laryngeal voice. It has begun to stabilize the action of the laryngeal system in building up the process of phonation and in forming the initial semantic connections between signals of the laryngeal system and the organism's physiological needs. The cry of a baby varies according to its internal and external circumstances and stimulation during the first few months after birth, varying according to such conditions as hunger, pain, discomfort and comfort.

The semantic function of laryngeal voice is realized to its fullest in the spontaneous expression of the child's basic needs by the time the child is six months old. Through this, the social function of speech as the means of communication between adults, and between child and adult, is established, beginning with communication between mother and child; therefore, the child who loses its hearing at six months of age cannot be placed in the same category as the child who lost its hearing when it was four months younger.

These few examples have been worked out to explain the necessity for a system of classification of hearing-impaired children which takes into account not only peripheral deafness but also the acoustic and linguistic experience acquired by the central nervous system prior to the occurrence of deafness.

Children who never had contact with sound, either in their prenatal or postnatal life, may be classified as Group A, whereas children who lost their hearing ability during the first two months of postnatal life may be labelled as Group B. The lack of identity between these two groups has already been pointed out, due to the experience of children of Group B with sound during the prenatal period and the first two months of the postnatal period, which established a network of relationships between sounds, the auditory system and the laryngeal system, along with a feedback control of laryngeal action by means of the central nervous system and the auditory system.

Children who lost their hearing during the prelingual period of postnatal life, between two and six months after birth, may be classified as Group C. In this group, only the meanings of laryngeal signals for purposes of communication will have been established. Between six months and twenty-four months, linguistic development of the normally hearing child is characterized by the formation of word meaning. In this period, laryngeal signals and expressions, based on the vibration of the vocal cords, begin to undergo a transformation to a qualitatively different system of signals produced by the articulatory organs, the system of speech sounds. Children who have lost their hearing ability during this period may be classified as Group D.

Between twenty-four months and four years of age, grammatical forms and categories are developed in the customary course of language acquisition. Children who lose their hearing during this period will have achieved a higher stage of language development than children who lost their hearing earlier in life. These children may be categorized as Group E, and they could be contrasted with children who lost their hearing between four and seven years, Group F, for whom grammatical forms and categories, vocabulary and speech sounds had all stabilized. Children who lose their hearing ability after seven years of age may be regarded as having established language prior to the loss of their hearing.

From the linguistic point of view, the above development of a classificatory system based on contact with language during the prelingual period is of crucial value because the prelingual period, which lasts up to six months of age, is the one in which the baby develops the expression of emotion through the laryngeal system. This system generates the meaningful signals which carry these emotions, and during this prelingual period, the child stablilizes this mode or form of communication. If further development of language in the child is stopped by the onset of deafness, all previously learned signals of linguistic value are very quickly forgotten.

Language may be divided broadly into two major categories. The first category is rather primitive and common to all animals; it is that part of language which is organized by the activity of the vocal cords using intensity and melody as two primary parameters in the construction of the system of communicatory signals. The second category comprises that part of human speech which is built up on the basis of the first part of language; it is exclusively and solely human, being a superstructure created by the configuration and alteration of the speech organs and the flow of the air stream acting upon laryngeal action. Conceptualized in this way, it is easy to understand why a child lacking the initial linguistic experience of using laryngeal voice has difficulty in attaining the higher stage of speech because it lacks the foundation for building speech sounds and ultimately phonemes as the linguistic units essential for the acoustic organization of word meaning itself.

The transition from emotional expression based on the laryngeal system to the acoustic organization of meaning in terms of speech sounds and ultimately phonemes bridges the gap between the lower, more primitive mode of communication and the higher, exclusively human mode of communication by means of word meaning.

The successive linguistic stages of experience of the normally hearing child in the course of language acquisition have special relevance for the child who has missed some or all of these stages due to deafness. Classification of children according to their hearing remnants has meaning only if the linguistic difficulties, due not only to the quantity and quality of damage to the auditory sense but also to the delimitation of the potentiality of acquiring successive stages of language in the normal sequence, are considered. For this reason, two children with approximately the same remnants of hearing, but possessing different foundations of linguistic experience due to the difference in age for onset of deafness, will achieve quite different speech habilitation levels during training despite similarities of physical and mental ability.

A comprehensive system of classification is needed for hearing-impaired children which takes into account their ability to perceive and comprehend speech sounds due to their linguistic experience as well as the extent and intensity of their peripheral deafness. Such a system of classification would also assist in understanding children's responses to selectively amplified speech signals which are sometimes unexpected in terms of the type of deafness or the type or pattern of amplification.

Selective acoustic amplification of speech permits the hearing-impaired child to come into contact with the quality of speech sounds and to master the discrepancies in perception between laryngeal voice and vowel formants or consonant noises. Through the mechanism of selective amplification, the acoustic superstructure of human speech may generate articulatory actions which converge upon a matching of perceived and articulated speech events.

To accomplish the generation of articulatory events aimed at matching of perceived and articulated speech sounds, children must be classified in terms of their auditory potential for speech habilitation as well as their linguistic experience. Children assumed to have no remnants of hearing can be classified as Group 0. Children who can perceive only functions of laryngeal voice at about three tone levels and a series of intensity levels based on the dynamics resulting from these tone levels comprise Group 1. Those children who are completely able to come into contact with the acoustic activity of laryngeal voice, and those qualitative elements of Speech sound quality may be perceived by children classified as Group 3, approximately up to 800 Hz or even up to 1000 Hz, belong to Group 2. Speech sound quality may be perceived by children classified as Group 3, when auditory remnants above 6000 Hz are not needed, only with selective acoustic amplification, avoiding the confusion that is produced by linear amplification. Those children who can be habilitated by means of linear amplification, or slightly modified linear amplification, within a range of approximately 25 dB, form Group 4.

The above classification of children according to their peripheral deafness separates them into two broad categories. The first broad category is composed of Groups 0 and 1, i.e. children who can only utilize the laryngeal system, that is, the suprasegmentals of speech, in speech habilitation. For Group 0, this is achieved by utilizing the visual and tactile senses. Not only the visual and tactile, but also the auditory, senses are utilized for Group 1. For the approximately 22 percent of hearing-impaired children falling in this first broad category, the instruments required for speech habilitation training include vibrators, intensity indicators, noise indicators and speech sound quality indicators. The second major category, comprising Groups 3 and 4 or approximately 53 percent of hearing-impaired children, requires training instruments of the acoustic type, such as the selective auditory filter amplifier, selectors and different group and individual amplifiers, only for the auditory sense. Between these two major categories, approximately 22 percent of the hearing-impaired children, those belonging to Group 2, are found who have characteristics of both categories. They do not belong exclusively to either major category, but since they possess the characteristics of both categories, require in speech habilitation all instruments appropriate for both categories.

Classification of children as just described in terms of remnants of hearing, together with findings from phonetic audiometry identifying the complex acoustic elements of speech which the children can individually hear, enables the teacher to program speech habilitation in terms of the utilization of existing remnants of hearing. While peripheral deafness, up to this time, cannot be altered, the ability to perceive speech sounds based on linguistic experience can be altered or modified during the process of speech habilitation.

If it is possible to provoke and stimulate the mechanism of linguistic creation by enlarging the potentiality for reconstruction of speech signals utilizing minimally perceived linguistic elements, a level of linguistic proficiency can be achieved which will be greater than that expected in terms of the physiological limits imposed by the remnants of hearing. It is this linguistic proficiency which is the major objective of the speech habilitation program for hearing-impaired children deafened before the acquisition of speech.

REFERENCES

Bessy, Michael R.: *The Kostić Methodology for Speech and Language Rehabilitation of Hearing-Impaired Children: Instrumentation, Psychological and Linguistic Principles.* University of Wisconsin-Superior, Department of Psychology. Psycholinguistic Series Volume II, 1972.

Das, Rhea S.: Phonetic audiometry: Theory and application. *The Silent World,* 5:32–36, 1970; *Govor i jezik kod lica sa oštećenim sluhom,* 5:1–6, 1971.

Kostić, Djordje, and Stošić, M.: *Akustička Struktura Krika Novorodenčeta* (The Acoustical Structure of the Cries of a New-born Infant). Belgrade, Institute for Experimental Phonetics and Speech Pathology. Report No. 10, EF-No. 3, 1963.

Kostić, Djordje, and Stošić, M.: *Akustiča Struktura Krika Odojceta Petnaestog Dana Po Rodenju* (The Acoustical Structure of the Cries of a Fifteen-day-old Infant). Belgrade, Institute for Experimental Phonetics and Speech Pathology, 1954.

Kostić, Djordje, Ilić, Č., Keramitčievski, S., Nikolić, M. and Kalic, D.D.: Fonetska audiometrija (Phonetic audiometry). *Defektologija, 2:*68–74, 1966. Phonetic audiometry. *Educational Miscellany, VI:*85–91, 1969.

Kostić, Djordje.: The integrated linguistic approach to the speech rehabilitation of deaf and hard-of-hearing children. *The Silent World, 5:*1–10, 1970.

Kostic, Djordje.: *Metodika Izgradnje Govora u Dece Ostećena Sluha* (Methodology of Speech Rehabilitation for Deaf and Hard-of-Hearing Children). Belgrade, Savez drustava defektologa Jugoslavije, 1971, 1–363.

Walton, Jane K.: *An Empirical Study of Hearing Impairment, Intelligence and Habilitation of Speech Utilizing the Kostić Methodology.* University of Wisconsin-Superior, Department of Psychology. Psycholinguistic Series Volume III, 1973.

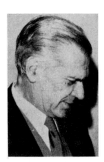

PROFESSOR DJORDJE KOSTIĆ

Professor Djordje Kostić, Yugoslav linguist and phonetician, founded the Institute for Experimental Phonetics and Speech Pathology (then the Institute for Experimental Phonetics, Speech Pathology, and Foreign Language Research) in 1953. Professor Kostić has been the Director of the Institute since its inception and following its reorganization in 1962. Prior to the founding of the Institute, he was chief of the Department of Experimental Phonetics within the Institute for Serbocroatian Language of the Serbian Academy of Science and Arts. His previous appointments include those of Professor of General and Experimental Phonetics, Faculty of Philosophy, University of Belgrade and Chief Editor, Foreign Language Broadcasts, Yugoslav Radio.

Professor Kostić was educated at the University of Belgrade, at the Sorbonne and at University College, London. In London he carried out postgraduate studies in general phonetics and English phonetics under the late Professor Daniel Jones. He has carried out research and published books and articles in the following areas of specialization: acoustic phonetics and phonology, grammatical structure, audiometry, speech habilitation of the hearing-impaired, adult literacy, foreign language teaching and multilingualism. He has published over one hundred articles and over twenty books in the Serbocroatian language, English language and other languages. He has visited a number of countries on governmental request as an expert, on study tour to collect technical information, in connection with scientific congresses and as guest professor. Since 1968, he has been Visiting Research Professor, Indian Statistical Institute, Calcutta, India, and since 1971, he has been on the Summer Faculty of the University of Wisconsin-Superior. He is a member of the Linguistic Society of America, the International Society of Audiologists and Phoneticians, the

European Linguistics Society, the Japanese Society for Phonetics and similar professional societies in Yugoslavia.

Professor Kostić has been associated, as director of a collaborating research center, with the Center for Comparative Psycholinguistics, University of Illinois, since 1964. He was Principal Investigator, Foreign Language Laboratory Project, United States Technical Aid, in Yugoslavia from 1956 to 1959. Currently he is Principal Investigator of two Indian Health Service (United States Public Health Service) research projects being conducted in Yugoslavia: 'Linguistic Habilitation of the Hearing-Impaired" and "Development and Evaluation of a Phonetic Audiometer Based upon the Navajo Language."

In his private life, he writes and publishes literary works, including books and poetry and also paints. Within the last five years, his paintings have been exhibited at the National Museum of Contemporary Art, Belgrade; the Academy of Fine Arts, Calcutta, India; the Museum of Decorative Arts, Palais du Louvre, Paris and have also been published in several books.

Chapter XX

A STUDY OF THE EFFECTS OF THE KOSTIĆ METHODOLOGY ON SPEECH SOUND QUALITY AND LARYNGEAL VOICE OF HEARING IMPAIRED CHILDREN

Rhea S. Das, Frances M. Kain and Jane K. Walton

In their 1973 review of aural rehabilitation, J.J. O'Neill and H.J. Dyer have stated:

> One of the future directions in aural rehabilitation research should be the elaboration of a conceptual framework to describe the process. Through this should emerge the constructs that are supported by extant scientific data and, likewise, the constructs that are not supported by scientific data. . . . Another direction for future research should be the shift in approach from one of primarily lip-reading and auditory training to a much broader approach that embraces language development, the social ramifications of hearing loss and also vocational aspects. (O'Neill and Oyer, 1973, p. 246).

Earlier, in the same review, they state that ". . . habilitative and rehabilitative procedures must be employed that make optimal use of the residual hearing of the handicapped individual." (O'Neill and Oyer, p. 232).

They also emphasize the necessity of developing specifications for amplification systems for the hearing handicapped, instead of adapting aural rehabilitation procedures to the specifications currently set by commercial sources.

A theoretical framework for the aural habilitation of hearing-impaired children which takes into account both the residual hearing of the handicapped individual and the necessity of developing an amplification system which provides selective amplification of sound according to the residual hearing of the handicapped children has been developed by Professor Djordje Kostić, Director of the Institute for Experimental Phonetics and Speech Pathology, Belgrade, Yugoslavia. Referred to as the Kostić Methodology, this theoretical framework is linguistic in conceptualization, and integrates auditory, phonetic and psychological principles to arrive at a teaching strategy appropriate for the type of hearing loss being treated. Four guiding principles are formulated by Kostić (1970, 1971) which provide the objectives of the teaching strategy. The first guiding principle concerns time or duration in human speech. During the prelingual period of life, the child with normal hearing orients himself or herself to the world of sound, its time, intensity and frequency. Since human speech is an event in time, it is necessary for the hearing-impaired child to develop a sense of acoustic time.

The second guiding principle places the development of the supra-segmentals of speech before the development of speech sounds because they are more general than speech sounds from a linguistic point of view. Since languages differ in their suprasegmental characteristics, the specific techniques and models must be worked out separately for each language. Stress or intensity, tone or word melody and duration or time of the laryngeal voice define the three major suprasegmentals.

The third guiding principle is that all speech factors must be combined, using special technical apparatus, in such a way that they will produce the same effect as speech factors for children with normal hearing. This combination of speech factors must follow the same sequence of language acquisition as experienced by the child with normal hearing. It also means that speech sounds must be interwoven in the suprasegmental frames characteristic of the language, not those learned in isolated positions, so that the natural acoustic structure emerges which organizes word meaning.

The fourth guiding principle calls for motivation of the learning process through utilization of meaningful actions, expresing the need of the child and at the same time the requirements imposed upon the child by the environment and individuals in that environment. Through this principle, the social function of language is developed in the child. These four guiding principles form one, unified theoretical framework which defines the habilitative methodology according to the residual hearing of the child, the age of onset of hearing loss and the age at which habilitation is initiated.

In terms of residual hearing, Kostić distinguishes five categories: 0, I, II, III and IV. Children lacking any identifiable residual hearing are classified as Group 0. Children whose residual hearing permits them only to perceive functions of laryngeal voice at about three tone levels and a series of intensity levels based on those tone levels are classified as Group I. Usually the residual hearing of Group I children is restricted to a small range of 100 Hz width or less. Children who are able to perceive the acoustic activity of laryngeal voice, and the acoustic quality of speech sounds within the range of larygneal voice, due to residual hearing extending up to 800Hz or even 1000 Hz are assigned to Group II. Children whose residual hearing extends from 1000 Hz to 3000 Hz, with intensity dynamics of 15 dB to 25 dB, are placed in Group III; these children can perceive

speech sound quality if they are provided with selective amplification according to their audiograms. Children for whom the audiogram is relatively linear, so that one portion of the frequency spectrum can be amplified to the same degree as all other portions of the frequency spectrum,
are classified as Group IV and can be habilitated using linear amplification
if their intensity dynamics have a range of 25 dB. A separate teaching
strategy has been formulated for each of these five groups of children,
which makes use of special apparatus developed by Kostić for the habilitation of the hearing-impaired.

The complete set of apparatus for the habilitation of the hearing-
impaired developed by Kostić is multisensory in configuration. Not only
the auditory sense, but also the visual and tactual senses of the child, are
stimulated by speech factors processed through these instruments. Highly
selective amplification of sound, adjusted to the audiometric threshold of
the child, is provided by the Selective Auditory Filter Amplifier, which
is composed of twenty-seven independent units, each of which processes
a segment of the frequency spectrum. The lowest unit begins at 95 Hz
and the highest unit ends at 14,354 Hz. Each unit can be adjusted separately in terms of intensity as well as 'Q' factor. The Selective Auditory
Filter Amplifier is used routinely for children of Groups I, II and III and
may also be used for special training of children in Group IV. Another
acoustic instrument designed to provide auditory input for the child is
the Selector. Selectors are provided in sets of eight, each Selector providing a different pattern of selective amplification within a limited intensity and dynamic range, suitable for habilitation of Group IV children.
Transformation of acoustic speech data into a form suitable for visual
input to the child is made possible by means of the Intensity Indicator,
the Friction Indicator and the Nasality Indicator. The Intensity Indicator
allows the child to adjust his voice so that it is neither too loud nor too
soft; it consists of a series of five light bulbs which light up according to
the intensity of microphone voice input. Since the fricative and affricate
consonants require generation of high frequency noise-like energy, the
Friction Indicator has been developed to provide a visual indication of
the intensity of those frequency regions relevant for these speech sounds.
The presence of nasality in speech sounds can be detected using the
Nasality Indicator, which provides visual input to the child regarding
acceptable nasalization, too little nasalization or too much nasalization.
In addition to the auditory and visual instruments, an instrument utilizing
the tactual sense for obtaining information about speech factors has been
developed by Kostić. Labelled 'Vibrators,' a vibrating membrane responding to laryngeal voice is placed on a box which the child then places its
fingers on. Two boxes are used per child, one for each hand. This instru-

ment permits the child to perceive variations in laryngeal voice, discrimination of voiced and voiceless consonants, duration of speech sounds, syllabic stress, the overall intensity pattern of speech, differences in pitch level, as well as elements distinguishing different categories of speech sounds. A more complete description of these instruments is provided by Bessy (1972).

The objective of aural rehabilitation in the Kostić Methodology is the linguistic development of the child, in which it is necessary first of all to establish the sensory and perceptual foundation of orally communicated language and then to develop the response patterns essential for oral communication, hence input and perception, followed by output or response. Through the use of special instruments, multisensory but emphasizing selective amplification of acoustic signals according to the audiogram of the hearing-impaired child and teaching strategies for the different categories of children (0, I, II, III and IV) based on the four guiding principles, habilitation is sought which has as its objective the development of oral language. The preliminary stages in the linguistic development sequence include control of laryngeal voice, development of suprasegmentals and development of speech sounds. To assess the progress of the child in its oral language acquisition, Kostić has devised a series of tests for evaluation of articulation. Based on phonetic principles and findings in speech pathology, these tests require the trained ear of the professional phonetician, speech therapist, speech pathologist or teacher of the deaf trained in speech. Evaluation of laryngeal voice, for example, calls for consideration of the tenseness, looseness, damping and frequency of usage of laryngeal voice. In evaluating speech sounds, the different categories of speech sounds, viz. vowels, diphthongs, plosives, affricates, fricatives, laterals and nasals, may be considered in terms of overall clarity of pronunciation, in terms of duration, nasalization, centralization and perceptual quality, or in even more diagnostic terms defining the locus and mode of articulation. This study will report changes in articulation resulting from training over a one month period utilizing the Kostić Methodology.

DESIGN OF THE STUDY

The Kostić Methodology was introduced concurrently at the university level for specialized training and at the public schools implementation level for habilitation of hearing-impaired children in a one month program, June 19 to July 14, 1972. The university level program was carried out by the Department of Psychology, University of Wisconsin-Superior, in a Summer Work Conference, "Psycholinguistic Methodology for the Speech and Language Rehabilitation of Hearing-Impaired Children," under the sponsorship of Professor Joseph J. DeLucia, Chairman, Department of Psychology. Consultants and faculty for the Summer Work Conference were Professor Djordje Kostić, Professor Rhea S. Das, Dr. Spasenija Vladisavljević, Mr. Michael Bessy and Ms. Jane K. Walton. The public schools level program was carried out under a Title IV Program, "Summer Enrichment for the Hearing-Impaired" at the Weisberg Memorial Center of the Superior Public Schools, of which Mr. Michael Verich is the superintendent. The program was carred out under the immediate guidance of Mr. Richard Ballou, Director of Special Services, and the Certified Teacher of the Deaf responsible for the training of the hearing-impaired children was Ms. Frances M. Kain. In addition to university, local, state and federal funding which made the programs possible, the assistance of Dr. Joseph L. Stewart, Communication Disorders Specialist, Medical Services Branch, Indian Health Service, in combining the efforts of the Public Law-480 Research Project "Linguistic Habilitation of the Hearing-Impaired" (Institute for Experimental Phonetics and Speech Pathology, Belgrade, Yugoslavia, Professor Djordje Kostić, Principal Investigator) with those of the university, was also essential in realization of the programs comprising the introduction of the Kostić Methodology to the United States.

Eleven children in the summer, hearing-impaired special program served as subjects for this study. All were children regularly enrolled in the special education (deaf) classes of the Superior Public Schools. Three children also enrolled in the program were excluded from this study, as they were over twelve years of age; an additional two children could not be included as they were absent during the final recording for evaluation of their posttraining speech.

Table XX-I summarizes the characteristics of the sample of eleven children serving as subjects for this study. They ranged in age from 81 months (6 years 9 months) to 131 months (10 years 11 months). Prior to the initiation of training under the Kostić Methodology, the following psychological tests were administered to each child: Leiter International Performance Scale (Leiter, 1952), Performance Tests of the Wechsler Intelligence Scale for Children (Wechsler, 1949), The Bender Gestalt Test for Young Children (Koppitz, 1964) and The Human Figure Drawing Test (Koppitz, 1968). These four tests will be referred to as the Leiter, WISC, Bender-Gestalt and HFD, respectively, in the rest of this report. The tests were scored according to their manuals, and results for the Leiter and WISC are expressed in terms of published chronological age norms for the normally hearing child. Raw scores on the Bender-Gestalt were converted to standard scores with a mean of 100 and a standard deviation of 15. Raw scores on the HFD were recorded without norms or transformations; they reflect indications of emotionality. Audiometric determinations of the absolute threshold were made using the Peters AP31 Diagnostic Audiometer using air conduction for the right and left ears at the following signals (Hz or cyles per second): 125, 250, 500, 750, 1000, 1500, 2000, 3000, 4000, 6000 and 8000. The range of the threshold values is reported in Table XX-I and presented graphically in Figure XX-1. The minimum threshold curves in Figure XX-1 describe the residual hearing profile typical of a Group III child (curves 1 and 2) and of a Group I child (curves 3 and 4). Standard audiometric procedure was adopted (J. O'Neill and Oyer, 1966).

Table XX-I

CHRONOLOGICAL AGE, PSYCHOLOGICAL TEST PERFORMANCE
AND AUDIOMETRIC CHARACTERISTICS OF THE SAMPLE
OF ELEVEN HEARING-IMPAIRED CHILDREN

Measured Characteristic		Range		Mean	Standard Deviation
		Minimum	Maximum		
Age in months		81	131	98.2	16.7
Leiter		59	113	89.5	15.3
WISC		75	121	100.7	14.1
Bender-Gestalt		82	120	99.3	12.3
Human Figure Drawing		3	9	5.1	1.6
Audiometric Thresholds					
Frequency	Ear				
125	R	20	*	70.0	29.1
	L	25	*	67.3	30.1
250	R	30	95	72.3	17.1
	L	35	100	75.0	16.9
500	R	30	110	84.5	21.8
	L	30	110	83.6	22.3
750	R	55	*	89.5	18.8
	L	25	*	88.2	27.0
1000	R	55	*	91.4	18.2
	L	55	*	94.5	22.0
1500	R	55	*	90.0	19.7
	L	70	*	94.5	17.8
2000	R	55	*	87.7	21.2
	L	65	*	97.3	20.4
3000	R	55	*	88.6	23.4
	L	55	*	92.7	25.0
4000	R	55	*	90.5	24.5
	L	50	*	95.5	26.8
6000	R	45	*	88.6	29.4
	L	35	*	94.5	29.4
8000	R	20	*	86.4	34.0
	L	20	*	95.0	33.4

*Audiometric threshold not reached at 120 dB amplification; value of 120 dB inserted for computation of means, standard deviations and all subsequent statistical analysis.

In addition to the observed maximum and minimun values observed for the sample of eleven children, Table XX-I also presents the means and standard deviations observed for the sample. For the audiometric determinations, failure to achieve a threshhold determination at 120 dB was treated numerically as a threshold of 120 dB for convenience in subsequent statistical calculations, as the possibility of some residual hear-

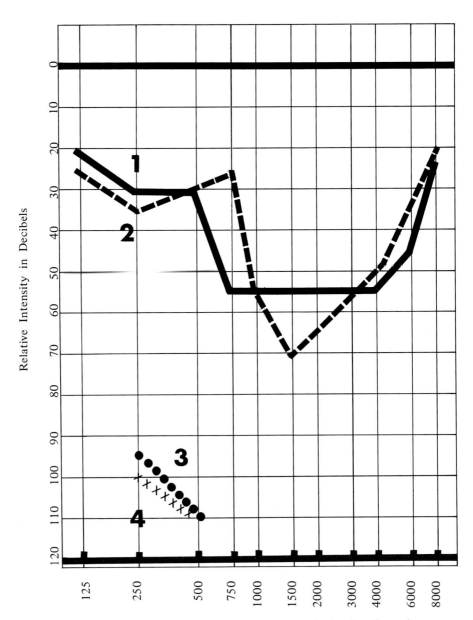

Frequency of Pure Tone Signal in Cycles Per Second

Figure XX-1. Minimum and maximum audiometric thresholds characterizing the sample of eleven hearing-impaired children. Code: (1) minimum threshold, right ear; (2) minimum threshold, left ear; (3) maximum threshold, right ear; (4) maximum threshold, left ear.

Table XX-II

MATRIX OF INTERCORRELATIONS FOR CHRONOLOGICAL
AGE AND PSYCHOLOGICAL TEST PERFORMANCE

	Leiter	WISC	Bender-Gestalt	Human Figure Drawing
Chronological Age	− 0.43	− 0.34	− 0.34	− 0.07
Leiter	----	0.72*	0.32	0.05
WISC		----	0.51	0.08
Bender-Gestalt			----	0.20

*Null hypothesis rejected, five percent level

ing at the asterisked frequencies could not be overruled. The relationships among the psychological tests are reported as coefficients of correlation in Table XX-II. A positive, significant correlation was obtained only between the WISC and the Leiter; these two tests both serve to estimate nonverbal general intelligence. The Bender-Gestalt and HFD were not significantly related to each other or to the other tests. The relationships among the audiometric determinations are presented in Table XX-III as coefficients of correlation. The highest coefficients of correlation occur in the cells next to the diagonal of the matrix of intercorrelations, which means that sensitivity to a given audiometric signal is most closely related to the sensitivity of an adjacent audiometric signal

Table XX-III

MATRIX OF INTERCORRELATIONS FOR AUDIOMETRIC
THRESHOLD DETERMINATIONS FOR THE RIGHT AND LEFT EAR*

Audiometric Signal and Ear		Frequency of Audiometric Signal									
		250	500	750	1000	1500	2000	3000	4000	6000	8000
125	R	0.76	0.68	0.51	0.31	0.27	0.31	0.22	0.21	− 0.01	0.06
	L	0.63	0.62	0.75	0.73	0.72	0.58	0.55	0.58	0.67	0.57
250	R	----	0.94	0.69	0.50	0.56	0.59	0.50	0.47	0.30	0.30
	L	----	0.96	0.94	0.86	0.71	0.66	0.53	0.56	0.54	0.42
500	R		----	0.79	0.61	0.63	0.65	0.60	0.60	0.42	0.45
	L		----	0.95	0.84	0.72	0.68	0.57	0.61	0.61	0.51
750	R			----	0.94	0.91	0.92	0.85	0.85	0.73	0.68
	L			----	0.91	0.83	0.76	0.65	0.68	0.67	0.58
1000	R				----	0.97	0.96	0.93	0.91	0.83	0.71
	L				----	0.86	0.84	0.72	0.77	0.81	0.74
1500	R					----	0.98	0.92	0.89	0.83	0.69
	L					----	0.93	0.86	0.90	0.86	0.77
2000	R						----	0.96	0.92	0.86	0.77
	L						----	0.96	0.95	0.92	0.87
3000	R							----	0.98	0.94	0.82
	L							----	0.98	0.91	0.86
4000	R								----	0.95	0.87
	L								----	0.93	0.88
6000	R									----	0.92
	L									----	0.97

*Reject null hypothesis at five percent level if correlation coefficient exceeds 0.60; at one percent level if coefficient exceeds 0.73.

(adjacent in the sense of frequency in Hz or cycles per second). If hearing loss were uniform throughout the frequency spectrum, then all coefficients of correlation in Table XX-III would be approximately equal. The presence of correlation coefficients significantly different from zero at the one percent and five percent levels and of correlation cofficients not differing significantly from zero, in the same matrix, rejects the hypothesis of uniform or linear hearing loss throughout the frequency spectrum for this sample of subjects.

In the week before initiation of training under the Kostić Methodology, Ms. Kain recorded the pronunciation of the children using the stimulus words of the Test for Screening Articulatory Defects in American English (Kostić, 1971, 1972). Using an Ampex Tape Recorder at 1¾ ips, Ms. Kain pronounced each stimulus word into a microphone, facing the child. She used no special signs or gestures for the deaf. The child repeated the word pronounced by Ms. Kain, and the child's pronunciation was also recorded. The children did not wear their hearing aids, so as to avoid the distortion upon their hearing introduced by the specifications of the hearing aids interacting with their residual hearing and, at the same time, to estimate their ability to perceive and repeat the words from auditory and visual input, i.e. at their base level. The stimulus words employed, chosen specifically for the North Central American English characteristic of northwestern Wisconsin pronunciation, and the speech sounds which they were used to evaluate, follow: feet (i:), lips (i), lake (e), met (ε), at (æ), ask (a), father (α), not (ɤ), all (ɔ:), obey (o), foot (u), boot (u:), up (Λ), bird (ɚ) and about (ə) for the vowels; say (ei), I (ai), boy (i), new (iu), out (au) and go (ou) for the diphthongs; pipe (p), best (b), tube (t), did (d), kick (k) and go (g) for the plosives; cats (ts), birds (dz), church (tʃ), judge (d₃), street (tr) and dream (dr) for the affricates; five (f), voice (v), thin (θ), this (ʒ), sea (s), zoo (z), she (ʃ), pleasure (ʒ), he (h), yellow (j), when (wh) and very (r) for the fricatives; lip (light l) and film (dark ł) for the lateral and melon (m), not (n) and thing (η) for the nasals. The pronunciation of each child was evaluated using parts (3) and (4) of the Test for Screening Articulatory Defects in American English (Kostić, 1971, 1972); the evaluation was made without knowledge of the child's audiogram or psychological test performance. Table XX-IV gives the maximum and minimum values of the evaluations for laryngeal voice (f_o) and the speech sound quality of vowels, diphthongs, plosives, affricates, fricatives, lateral and nasals, for the pronunciation of the children in the pretraining recording session. Means and standard deviations are also presented in Table XX-IV. The detailed data are reported in Walton (1973).

Training of the children according to the Kostić Methodology was

Table XX-IV

EVALUATIONS OF PRETRAINING AND POSTTRAINING LARYNGEAL
VOICE (f_0)* AND SPEECH SOUND QUALITY OF ELEVEN HEARING-IMPAIRED
CHILDREN

Evaluation	Range		Mean	Standard Deviation
	Minimum	Maximum		
Pretraining				
f_0	0	8.0	4.5	2.3
Vowels	2.1	7.0	4.9	1.9
Diphthongs	1.8	7.0	5.1	2.0
Plosives	2.0	7.0	5.1	1.9
Affricates	1.5	7.0	5.7	2.0
Fricatives	2.0	7.0	5.7	1.9
Lateral and Nasals	2.6	7.0	5.6	1.7
Posttraining				
f_0	0	5.0	1.1	1.6
Vowels	1.0	7.0	3.6	2.2
Diphthongs	1.0	7.0	3.7	2.5
Plosives	1.0	7.0	3.5	2.2
Affricates	1.2	7.0	4.9	2.3
Fricatives	1.4	7.0	4.4	2.2
Lateral and Nasals	1.0	7.0	4.4	2.7

*Kostić, Dj.: Test for Screening Articulatory Defects in American English: Quality and Usage of Laryngeal Voice. A value of 0 indicates correct quality and usage of f_0; increasing values indicate increasingly poor f_0.

**Kostić, Dj.: Test for Screening Articulatory Defects in American English: Rating of Overall Characteristics of Speech Sounds. A value of 1 indicates clear, undistorted pronunciation and a value of 7 indicates completely distorted pronunciation.

carried out on an individual basis daily, five days a week, during the one month period from June 19 to July 14, 1972. The children were trained by Ms. Kain utilizing the following special equipment: Selective Audidtory Filter Amplifier, Selectors, Intensity Indicator and Vibrators. Each child received approximately fifteen minutes of training each day. The methodology employed has been reported in detail elsewhere (Kostić, 1971, in the Serbocroatian language; Kostić, Das, and Mitter, in press, written in the English language for habilitation of the Bengali language).

On the final two days of the one-month training period, the pronunciation of the children in response to the stimulus words used in the pretraining test of articulation was again recorded. The procedure employed was identical to that of the pretraining recording session with one exception: each child received the auditory stimulus through headphones connected to the Selective Auditory Filter Amplifier adjusted to compensate for the child's hearing loss to the extent possible (i.e. selective or nonlinear amplification according to the child's audiogram). Ms. Kain pronounced the words through the microphone connected to the Selective Auditory Filter Amplifier, facing the child and using no special signs or gestures for the deaf. The child also spoke into the microphone and could therefore hear his or her own response, according to the same pattern of amplification. The pronunciation both of Ms. Kain and the children was recorded on the Ampex Tape Recorder. The posttraining evaluation of laryngeal voice and speech sound quality was carried out in the same manner as for the pretraining evaluation. The results are summarized in Table XX-IV, which gives the minimum and maximum values, means and standard deviations.

RESULTS OF THE STUDY

Relationships among the different categories of speech sounds, and their relationships to laryngeal voice, are summarized as coefficients of correlation in Tables XX-V and XX-VI. Table XX-V, dealing with pretraining evaluations of speech sounds and laryngeal voice, shows statistically significant relationships among all categories of speech sounds and between laryngeal voice and all categories of speech sounds except fricatives. This indicates that children who have better pronunciation for any one category of speech sounds will tend to have better pronunciation for all other categories as well as for laryngeal voice. The latter relationship indicates that control of laryngeal voice is not separate from pronunciation of speech sounds, that is, a child tends to be fairly good or fairly poor on all of these measures. In the posttraining situation, the degree of interrelationship among the different categories of speech sounds remains significantly high; however, as Table XX-VI shows, the degree of relationship between laryngeal voice and the different categories of speech sounds is changed. This occurs because children who were previously poor both in control of laryngeal voice and in speech sound pronunciation have improved in their control of laryngeal voice during the first month of training to a greater extent than they have improved in their pronunciation of speech sounds. This is shown by Table XX-VII, where the pretraining and posttraining means are compared. Whereas a change of 3.4 points occurred for laryngeal voice, the change in speech sound evaluations ranged from 0.8 to 1.6 points. As the development of laryngeal voice and its dynamics, including the suprasegmentals, is one of the initial objectives of the Kostić Methodology, this finding may be regarded as supportive of the theory.

The basic question posed in this study was whether or not training for a one-month period utilizing the Kostić Methodology would significantly affect the pronunciation of hearing-impaired children. Comparing the pretraining and posttraining evaluations of laryngeal voice and of speech sound quality by means of Wilcoxon's Test for Paired Comparisons (McCall, 1970) yields an affirmative answer. The changes are statistically significant at either the 5 percent or 1 percent levels for laryngeal voice and the different categories of speech sounds, as shown in Table XX-VII. Having confirmed the possibility of change, even in such a short period

Table XX-V

MATRIX OF INTERCORRELATIONS FOR EVALUATIONS OF
PRETRAINING LARYNGEAL VOICE AND SPEECH SOUND QUALITY

	Vowels	Diphthongs	Plosives	Affricates	Fricatives	Lateral and Nasals
Laryngeal Voice (f_0)	0.61*	0.61*	0.74**	0.63*	0.48	0.69*
Vowels	----	0.96**	0.94**	0.83**	0.85**	0.92**
Diphthongs		----	0.90**	0.77**	0.81**	0.85**
Plosives			----	0.98**	0.82**	0.94**
Affricates				----	0.95**	0.97**
Fricatives					----	0.95**

*Null hypothesis rejected; five percent level.
**Null hypothesis rejected, one percent level.

Table XX-VI

MATRIX OF INTERCORRELATIONS FOR EVALUATIONS OF
POSTTRAINING LARYNGEAL VOICE AND SPEECH SOUND QUALITY

	Vowels	Diphthongs	Plosives	Affricates	Fricatives	Lateral and Nasals
Laryngeal Voice (f_0)	0.80**	0.64**	0.69*	0.57	0.52	0.54
Vowels	----	0.93**	0.92**	0.88**	0.86**	0.92**
Diphthongs		----	0.92**	0.89**	0.88**	0.88**
Plosives			----	0.82**	0.76**	0.85**
Affricates				----	0.88**	0.88**
Fricatives					----	0.91**

*Null hypothesis rejected, five percent level.
**Null hypothesis rejected, one percent level.

Table XX-VII

STATISTICAL COMPARISON OF PRETRAINING AND POSTTRAINING
EVALUATIONS OF LARYNGEAL VOICE AND SPEECH SOUND QUALITY

Evaluation	Mean Pretraining	Mean Posttraining	Change	W*	Significance
Laryngeal Voice	4.5	1.1	3.4	0	1%
Vowels	4.9	3.6	1.3	1	1%
Diphthongs	5.1	3.7	1.4	0	1%
Plosives	5.1	3.5	1.6	0	1%
Affricates	5.7	4.9	0.8	0	1%
Fricatives	5.7	4.4	1.3	0	1%
Lateral and Nasals	5.6	4.4	1.2	5	5%

*Wilcoxon's Test for Paired Comparisons; significance indicates level of rejection of null hypothesis.

of training under the Kostić Methodology, the next question which arises is the relationship of psychological test performance and the pattern of residual hearing to quality of laryngeal voice and of speech sounds.

To answer the second question posed in this study, the relationship of psychological test performance and of residual hearing to pronunciation, multiple regression analysis was carried out (Chakravarti, Laha and Roy, 1967). The stepwise method of multiple regression analysis developed by M.A. Efroymson (Ralston and Wilf, 1960) was adopted, in which only those variables are included in the final equation which are statistically significant, i.e. they contribue at a specified level of significance to the *goodness of fit* of the equation to the observed data. The calculations were carried out on the University of Wisconsin-Superior Data Processing Center's IBM 1130 Computing System, using the IBM 1130 Statistical System Program (IBM, 1970). The essential results of this statistical analysis are presented in Tables XX-VIII to XX-XIV for posttraining laryngeal voice, vowel quality, diphthong quality, plosive quality, affricate quality, fricative quality and lateral and nasal quality.

Considering prediction of posttraining f_o or laryngeal voice first, Table XX-VIII may be examined. Coefficients of correlation express the relationship of each measured characteristic (age, psychological test, audiometric determination) to the evaluation of posttraining f_o. Coefficients for age and psychological tests are entered under 'Right Ear' for convenience in presentation. The standard partial regression coefficients permit prediction of f_o given these measured characteristics, when both characteristics (age, psychological test, audiometric determination) and criterion (posttraining f_o) are expressed as normal deviates with a mean of zero and a standard deviation of one. The effect of all other variables on the relationship between each predictor (or measured characteristic) and the criterion has been parceled out, and only statistically significant predictor variables are retained. The relative size of the standard partial regression coefficients indicates their relative importance in predicting the criterion. For prediction of f_o, the most important variables are the audiometric determinations at 6000 and 8000 Hz for the right ear and the audiometric determination at 750 Hz for the left ear. The coefficients of the multiple repression equations are expressed in the units of measurement of the predictor variables, thus, in dB for the audiometric determinations. Use of the coefficients of the multiple regression equation permits prediction of the posttraining f_o, entering the observed values of the psychological tests and the observed dB values of the audiometric thresholds and adding (or subtracting) the appropriate fitted constant.

For prediction of posttraining f_o, three psychological tests are significant: Leiter, Bender-Gestalt and HFD. Audiometric thresholds at 125 Hz, 250 Hz, 500 Hz and 6000 Hz contribute significantly to the prediction of posttraining f_o. As shown in Table XX-IX, posttraining vowel quality is predicted from the Leiter and the WISC and audiometric thresholds at 2000 Hz and 8000 Hz for both ears. Other audiometric thresholds enter differentially into the equations for the right and left ears.

A similar predictive pattern is found for posttraining diphthong quality, as shown in Table XX-X, which is hardly surprising in terms of the fundamental phonetic similarities between vowels and diphthongs. For posttraining plosive quality, the Leiter and the Bender-Gestalt are the most important psychological test predictors, while audiometric thresholds at 750 Hz, 3000 Hz, 4000 Hz and 8000 Hz are the most important components of residual hearing for prediction. The importance of these audiometric

Table XX-VIII
PREDICTION OF POSTTRAINING f_0

Measured Characteristic	Correlations Right Ear	Correlations Left Ear	Standard Partial Regression Coefficients* Right Ear	Standard Partial Regression Coefficients* Left Ear	Multiple Regression Equations* Right Ear	Multiple Regression Equations* Left Ear
Chronological Age	—0.20					
Leiter	—0.10		—0.20	—0.09	—0.02	—0.01
WISC	—0.12					
Bender-Gestalt	—0.11		0.70	—0.50	0.09	—0.07
HFD	0.78		0.95	0.87	0.95	0.87
Audiometry						
125	0.05	0.63	0.47	0.30	0.03	0.02
250	0.51	0.58	—1.12	0.14	—0.11	0.01
500	0.46	0.46	0.81	—0.70	0.06	—0.05
750	0.57	0.50		1.33		0.08
1000	0.65	0.64		—0.67		—0.05
1500	0.76	0.55				
2000	0.77	0.55				
3000	0.78	0.54	4.07		0.28	
4000	0.67	0.49	—1.82		—0.12	
6000	0.70	0.55	—2.13	0.12	—0.12	0.01
Constant					—14.00	3.36

*In Tables XX-VIII to XX-XIV, standard partial regression coefficients and regression coefficients for the multiple regression equation are given only for variables entering the equation at the one percent level. Variables are removed from the equation at the 0.5 percent level. For each of these tables, the multiple correlation coefficient has been + 0.99 and the F ratio testing the significance of the multiple regression has reached the one percent point.

Table XX-IX
PREDICTION OF POSTTRAINING VOWEL QUALITY

Measured Characteristic	Correlations Right Ear	Correlations Left Ear	Standard Partial Regression Coefficients Right Ear	Standard Partial Regression Coefficients Left Ear	Multiple Regression Equations Right Ear	Multiple Regression Equations Left Ear
Chronological Age	—0.39		—0.36		—0.05	
Leiter	—0.27		—0.48	—1.07	—0.07	—0.15
WISC	—0.18		0.27	0.37	0.04	0.06
Bender-Gestalt	—0.68			—0.56		—0.10
HFD	0.40			—0.05		—0.06
Audiometry						
125	0.36	0.74		0.61		0.04
250	0.56	0.54	0.20		0.03	
500	0.58	0.50		0.69		0.07
750	0.84	0.56	—0.22		—0.03	
1000	0.90	0.56				
1500	0.93	0.49				
2000	0.93	0.52	0.18	0.64	0.02	0.07
3000	0.92	0.64	0.88		0.08	
4000	0.86	0.60	0.12		0.01	
6000	0.83	0.58		—2.64		—0.19
8000	0.68	0.49	—0.35	2.35	—0.02	0.15
Constant					2.55	10.37

Table XX-X
PREDICTION OF POSTTRAINING DIPHTHONG QUALITY

Measured Characteristic	Correlations Right Ear	Correlations Left Ear	Standard Partial Regression Coefficients Right Ear	Standard Partial Regression Coefficients Left Ear	Multiple Regression Equations Right Ear	Multiple Regression Equations Left Ear
Chronological Age	—0.39		—0.36		—0.05	
Leiter	—0.27		—0.48	—1.07	—0.07	—0.15
WISC	—0.18		0.27	0.37	0.04	0.06
Bender-Gestalt	—0.68			—0.56		—0.10
HFD	0.40			—0.05		—0.06
Audiometry						
125	0.05	0.63	0.47	0.30	0.03	0.02
125	0.36	0.74		0.61		0.04
250	0.56	0.54	0.20		0.03	
500	0.58	0.50		0.69		0.07
750	0.84	0.56	—0.22		—0.03	
1000	0.90	0.56				
1500	0.93	0.49				
2000	0.93	0.52	0.18	0.64	0.02	0.07
3000	0.92	0.64	0.88		0.08	
4000	0.86	0.60	0.12		0.01	
6000	0.83	0.58		—2.64		—0.19
8000	0.68	0.49	—0.35	2.35	—0.02	0.15
Constant					2.55	10.37

thresholds can be understood in terms of the acoustic pattern of plosive consonants.

A somewhat different picture emerges for posttraining affricate quality. Table XX-XII for affricates may be compared with Table XX-XI for plosives. For affricates, the Bender-Gestalt is the most significant psychological test, while audiometric thresholds at 750 Hz, 4000 Hz and 8000 Hz are significant predictors. The threshold for 3000 Hz has been dropped from the predictive equation for affricates, though it was found in the predictive equation for plosives.

In Table XX-XIII, a similar analysis of the data for posttraining fricative quality yields the following significant variables: chronological age and audiometric thresholds at 125 Hz, 250 Hz, 750 Hz and 1000 Hz. Consideration of the lateral and nasals, presented in Table XX-XIV, shows that chronological age, the Leiter and the WISC, along with thresholds at 125 Hz and 250Hz, are the significant predictors. The importance of the low frequencies, near laryngeal voice, is shown for f_o, affricates, fricatives and lateral and nasals. Mid spectrum thresholds are important for vowel quality and diphthong quality (e.g. at 2000 Hz), while higher spectrum thresholds (e.g. 3000 Hz and 4000 Hz) seem to be important for plosive and affricate quality.

DISCUSSION

It was pointed out earlier in this paper that the Kostić Methodology takes into account residual hearing and selective amplification defined by

Table XX-XI
PREDICTION OF POSTTRAINING PLOSIVE QUALITY

Measured Characteristic	Correlations		Standard Partial Regression Coefficients		Multiple Regression Equations	
	Right Ear	Left Ear	Right Ear	Left Ear	Right Ear	Left Ear
Chronological Age	—0.39			0.02		0.00
Leiter	—0.15		—0.17	—1.01	—0.02	—0.15
WISC	—0.15					
Bender-Gestalt	0.51		0.63	—0.12	0.11	—0.02
HFD	0.37			—0.24		—0.32
Audiometry						
125	0.48	0.70	0.93		0.07	
250	0.64	0.70				
500	0.61	0.70		1.57		0.15
750	0.72	0.67	—1.11	—0.27	—0.13	—0.02
1000	0.74	0.60				
1500	0.79	0.55	0.76		0.08	
2000	0.79	0.57				
3000	0.80	0.66	1.48	0.88	0.14	0.08
4000	0.78	0.65	—0.60	—1.62	—0.05	—0.13
6000	0.74	0.60	0.27		0.02	
8000	0.59	0.48	—0.39	1.05	—0.02	0.07
				Constant	—13.50	8.05

the pattern of residual hearing. It introduces between these two factors a third factor, the acoustic properties of laryngeal voice and of speech sounds. All three factors are considered in carrying out diagnosis of the hearing handicap and classification of the child according to its residual hearing, the teaching strategy to be employed together with the special instruments required and the evaluation of the child's linguistic develop-

Table XX-XII
PREDICTION OF POSTTRAINING AFFRICATE QUALITY

Measured Characteristic	Correlations		Standard Partial Regression Coefficients		Multiple Regression Equations	
	Right Ear	Left Ear	Right Ear	Left Ear	Right Ear	Left Ear
Chronological Age	—0.39					
Leiter	—0.76					
WISC	—0.29					
Bender-Gestalt	—0.11		—0.16	—0.36	—0.03	—0.07
HFD	0.19		—0.12		—0.17	
Audiometry						
125	0.56	0.68	0.49	0.81	0.04	0.06
250	0.61	0.46	—0.06	—0.49	—0.01	—0.07
500	0.69	0.49				
750	0.89	0.52	0.10	1.33	0.01	0.11
1000	0.89	0.51		—0.21		—0.02
1500	0.84	0.31		—1.96		—0.26
2000	0.89	0.35				
3000	0.89	0.46	0.15		0.01	
4000	0.88	0.45	—0.41	1.39	—0.04	0.12
6000	0.81	0.49	0.91		0.07	
8000	0.79	0.46	0.21	0.06	0.01	0.00
				Constant	0.09	16.68

Table XX-XIII
PREDICTION OF POSTTRAINING FRICATIVE QUALITY

Measured Characteristic	Correlations		Standard Partial Regression Coefficients		Multiple Regression Equations	
	Right Ear	Left Ear	Right Ear	Left Ear	Right Ear	Left Ear
Chronological Age	—0.61		—0.37	—1.09	—0.05	—0.14
Leiter	—0.13			—1.28		—0.19
WISC	—0.11			0.21		0.03
Bender-Gestalt	—0.13			—0.09		—0.02
HFD	0.14		0.20		0.27	
Audiometry						
125	0.59	0.55	0.57	—0.48	0.04	—0.04
250	0.58	0.40	—0.41	—0.85	—0.05	—0.11
500	0.57	0.43	0.06		0.01	
750	0.86	0.45	—0.32	1.39	—0.04	0.11
1000	0.83	0.37	0.97	1.50	0.12	0.15
1500	0.82	0.29		—1.39		—0.17
2000	0.86	0.34	0.61		0.06	
3000	0.73	0.47	—0.61		—0.06	
4000	0.70	0.43				
6000	0.63	0.39				
8000	0.61	0.37				
			Constant		0.06	36.32

ment. The findings reported in Tables XX-VIII to XX-XIV indicate a differential patterning of significant audiometric thresholds in the prediction of laryngeal voice and of different categories of speech sounds. This points to an inadequacy of pure tone audiometry. While pure tone audiometry is language-free, the signals do not reflect the complex frequency and intensity patterns to which an individual must be sensitive to perceive the correct quality of speech sounds. If the speech sound structure of

Table XX-XIV
PREDICTION OF POSTTRAINING LATERAL AND NASAL QUALITY

Measured Characteristic	Correlations		Standard Partial Regression Coefficients		Multiple Regression Equations	
	Right Ear	Left Ear	Right Ear	Left Ear	Right Ear	Left Ear
Chronological Age	—0.47		—0.48	—1.70	—0.08	—0.27
Leiter	—0.36		—0.75	—2.92	—0.13	—0.51
WISC	—0.17		0.29	0.99	0.06	0.19
Bender-Gestalt	—0.12			0.59		0.13
HFD	0.13					
Audiometry						
125	0.50	0.65	0.40	—1.59	0.04	—0.14
250	0.43	0.34	—0.07	—0.29	—0.01	—0.05
500	0.45	0.36		—0.13		—0.02
750	0.78	0.38	—0.12		—0.02	
1000	0.82	0.30		4.38		0.54
1500	0.78	0.31	—0.07		—0.01	
2000	0.79	0.30		—2.65		—0.35
3000	0.76	0.47	0.82		0.09	
4000	0.72	0.45				
6000	0.69	0.42	—0.14		—0.01	
8000	0.58	0.34				
			Constant		11.55	43.09

a language is considered, looking for similarities among acoustic patterns in speech sounds rather than differences, a series of audiometric signals can be developed which reflect the phonetic structure of the language. This concept, developed by Kostić and demonstrated for the Serbocroatian language (Kostić, et al., 1969; Das, 1970, 1971), is used for diagnosis and classification of children in the Kostić Methodology; it is called *phonetic audiometry*. Since the pure tones of conventional pure tone audiometry do not reflect the acoustic characteristics of speech sounds, they are inadequate as a basis for diagnosis and habilitation; phonetic audiometry, on the contrary, provides directly meaningful results, i.e. can the child hear the acoustic components required for diphthong perception or plosive perception. As yet, a phonetic audiometry for American English has not been developed; however, under a Public Law 480 research project, Professor Kostić is developing a phonetic audiometry for the Navajo language to be utilized by the Indian Health Service at its center at the University of New Mexico in Albuquerque. The results of this study suggest that improved diagnosis and classification of children may be possible if improvements or changes in audiometric signals take place. It may be mentioned that speech audiometry depends upon knowledge of language and hence is insufficient for the congenitally deaf who lack linguistic development.

A number of the points raised in considering the results of this study have been dealt with by Bilger (1973). The need for selective amplification, according to the individual audiogram, is underlined by Bilger's emphasis on nonlinearity of the ear (Bilger, 1973, pp. 486–487). The role of auditory perception in language development is convincingly described by Bilger, who concludes discussion on this problem with the statement:

> For those who sincerely doubt that the auditory system is necessary to speaking and to understanding speech and language, the plight of the congenitally deaf is cited as mute testimony to its significance. (Bilger, 1973, p. 484).

Regarding the inadequacy of pure tone audiometry for understanding speech perception, Bilger states that one of the major impediments to the acquisition of relevant data has been the assumption that ". . . pure tones are a sufficient stimulus." (Bilger, 1973, p. 484).

In concluding this discussion, it may be desirable to consider the long-range objective of aural rehabilitation. This is perhaps not the acquisition of language in and of itself, but the development of cognitive skills which will enable the hearing-impaired individual to adjust socially and vocationally in a society in which the cognitive capabilities associated with normal hearing are essential. The acquisition of language is not only important in providing the means of communication but also in developing and shaping the cognitive processes. The crucial role of auditory processes in structuring cognition has apparently not only been ignored by psychologists but also by audiologists. To again quote Bilger:

> The most obvious consequence of limiting the scope of audiology to perceptual phenomena is seen in terms of the general lack of success experienced by those who are willing to try to educate the deaf and rehabilitate the hard-of-hearing. The only information our perceptually-based audiology can offer to them is to suggest they make sounds louder. Audiological research probably could, by studying the role of audition in the context of memory, learning, decision making, etc., provide these educators with the information they need to do their work more effectively. (Bilger, 1973, pp. 484–485).

The Kostić Methodology, integrating audiology, phonetics and linguistics, and psychology, in the diagnosis, habilitation and evaluation of linguistic development in the hearing-impaired, may serve not only to provide a needed conceptual framework for aural rehabilitation but also to initiate and organize research on the role of auditory processes in structuring cognition through perception of language.

REFERENCES

Bessy, M.R.: The Kostić methodology for speech and language rehabilitation of hearing-impaired children: Instrumentation, psychological and linguistic principles. *Psycholinguistic Series, Volume II.* Department of Psychology, University of Wisconsin-Superior, 1972.

Bilger, R.C.: Research Frontiers in Audiology. In Jerger, J. (Ed.): *Modern Developments in Audiology,* 2nd ed. New York: Academic Press, 1973, pages 469–501.

Chakravarti, I.M.: Laha, R.G. and Roy, J.: *Handbook of Methods of Applied Statistics,* volume I. New York: John Wiley, 1967.

Das, R.S.: Phonetic audiometry: theory and application. *The Silent World,* 5:32–36; 1970, *Govor i jezik kod lica sa oštećenim sluhom,* 5:1–6, 1971.

IBM Application Program 1130 Statistical System (1130–CA–06X). Edition H20–0341–1. White Plains: International Business Machines Corporation, 1970.

Koppitz, E.M.: *The Bender Gestalt Test for Young Children.* New York: Grune and Stratton, 1964.

Koppitz, E.M.: *Psychological Evaluation of Children's Human Figure Drawings.* New York: Grune and Stratton, 1968.

Kostić, Dj.: The integrated linguistic approach to the speech rehabilitation of deaf and hard-of-hearing children. *The Silent World,* 5:1–10, 1970.

Kostić, Dj.: *Metodika izoradnje govora u dece oštećena sluha.* (Methodology of speech rehabilitation for deaf and hard-of-hearing children.) Belgrade: Savez drustava defektologa Jugosavije, 1971.

Kostić, Dj.: Test for Screening Articulatory Defects in American English: (1) Preliminary Screening; (2) Detailed Description; (3) Quality and Usage of Laryngeal Voice; and (4) Rating of Overall Characteristics of Speech Sounds. Department of Psychology, University of Wisconsin-Superior, 1971–1972.

Kostić, Dj.; Ilić, C.; Keramitčievski, S.; Nikolić, M. and Kalić, D.D.: Phonetic audiometry. (Translated by A. Mitter.) Education Directorate, Government of Tripura, *Educational Miscellany*, 6:85–91, 1969.

Kostić, Dj.; Das, R.S.; and Mitter, A.: *Bengali Speech Sounds for Deaf and Hard-of-Hearing Children*. Agartala, Tripura, India: Education Directorate, Government of Tripura (in press).

Leiter, R.G.: *Leiter International Performance Scale*. Chicago: C.H. Stoelting, 1952.

McCall, R.B.: *Fundamental Statistics for Psychology*. New York: Harcourt, Brace and World, 1970.

O'Neill, J. and Oyer, H.J.: *Applied Audiometry*. New York: Dodd, Mead, 1966.

O'Neill, J.J. and Oyer, H.J.: Aural rehabilitation. In Jerger, J. (Ed.): *Modern Developments in Audiology*, 2nd ed. New York: Academic Press, 1973. Pages 211–252.

Ralston, A. and Wilf, H.S.: *Mathematical Methods for Digital Computers*, volume I. New York: John Wiley, 1960.

Walton, J.K.: An empirical study of hearing impairment, intelligence and habilitation of speech utilizing the Kostić Methodology. *Psycholinguistic Series, Volume III*. Department of Psychology, University of Wisconsin-Superior, 1973.

Wechsler, D.: *Wechsler Intelligence Scale for Children*. New York: Psychological Corporation, 1949.

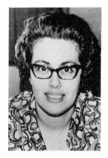

RHEA S. DAS, Ph.D.

Dr. Rhea S. Das has received her B.A. in major zoology in Illinois in 1951 with minors in chemistry and physiology. She received her M.A., majoring in psychology from Illinois in 1953 and her Ph.D. in social psychology with a minor in anthropology from Illinois in 1955.

HONORARY SOCIETIES
Sigma Xi, Phi Sigma

ASSISTANTSHIPS AND FELLOWSHIPS
Research and Teaching Assistantships.
University of Illinois, 1952–1955
Research Fellow, Indian Statistical Institute
for advanced study in England, October 1955-April 1956

EMPLOYMENT HISTORY
Professor, Department of Psychology, Wisconsin State University, Superior, Wisconsin 54880

Past: Professor and Director of Psycholinguistic and Psychometric Research, Indian Statistical Institute, Calcutta, India, 1962–1970; Visiting Associate Professor of Behavioral Science, Operations Research Group, Case Institute of Technology, Cleveland, Ohio, 1961–1962; Research Associate (Computer Programming), Psychophysiology Laboratory, Lafayette Clinic, Detroit, Michigan, 1960–1961; Research Associate, Department of Reading and Study Skills, Wayne State University, Detroit, Michigan, Summer 1966; Assistant Professor, Industrial Psychology and Psychometrics, Indian Statistical Institute, Calcutta, India, 1956–1960

EDITORIAL BOARD MEMBERSHIPS
Indian Journal of Applied Psychology, Indian Psychological Review, Indian Journal of Psychology

RESEARCH INTERESTS
Psycholinguistics (Linguistics, Cognition, Speech and Hearing); Psychometric Theory and Psychological Measurement; Statistical Studies in Psychology, Phonetics, Phonology, and Linguistics

RESEARCH PROJECTS
Research Collaborator with Charles E. Osgood, Center for Comparative Psycholinguistics Institute of Communications Research, University of Illinois, in the International Project on the Cross-Cultural Generality of Affective Meaning Systems

Research Collaborator with Djordje Kostić, Institute for Experimental Phonetics and Speech Pathology, Belgrade, Yugoslavia, in the area of Psycholinguistics, Phonetics, statistical and applied linguistics

Principal Investigator, U.S. Public Health Service Project on "Estimates of probabilities of hospitalization according to age, sex and diagnosis, and their use in planning hospital services," conducted at the Indian Statistical Institute, Calcutta, India

Chapter XXI

TEACHERS' OBSERVATION ON
THE RESULTS OF THE KOSTIĆ METHODOLOGY

FRANCES M. KAIN

EVALUATION OF EQUIPMENT FROM YUGOSLAVIA

ONE OF THE primary objectives of the summer school program in deaf education was to evalulate the effectiveness of equipment originated and designed by Professor Djordje Kostić and produced at the Institute for Experimental Phonetics and Speech Pathology, Belgrade, Yugoslavia. Through fundings by Title VI, state and local effort, a program was developed to determine the feasibility of this equipment for use in deaf education in the Superior Public Schools and ultimately for instruction in deaf education throughout the state of Wisconsin.

This equipment was available on loan for our use during the four-week period from June 19 through July 14, 1972, and during that time, all or parts of the equipment were in use every day. Miss Fran Kain, teacher of the hearing-impaired, was instructed in the use of the equipment and worked with the same children during this period of time. Four weeks is, in reality, too short a time for a comprehensive evaluation, though Miss Kain did record her observations on each piece of equipment. These observations, and recommendations on the basis of her observations, are found below on the following pieces of equipment: selective auditory filter amplifier, the vibrator, intensity indicator and selector.

SELECTIVE AUDITORY FILTER AMPLIFIER: (FILTER) The claim of this equipment is that through use of the filter, it is possible to amplify only those frequencies that the child needs to have amplified and only to the level needed. Prior to work on the filter, each child was given an audiometric examination. This latest audiogram was then used as a basis for amplification on the filter. The results indicated that fifteen children worked daily with the filter, and all fifteen were able to produce better speech sounds when using the filter. Eight of the children learned to articulate difficult speech sounds for the first time—such as the "s" and "t" sound and "k" or "g" sound. This was possible because of the selective

203

amplification but equally because through the filter, it is possible to *peak* or intensify each particular speech sound in question.

VIBRATOR: The vibrator is a device to transform voice into vibration by use of a microphone, an auditory filter, amplifier and the vibrator apparatus. The results indicated that for the fifteen children who used this vibrator, favorable results were obtained by all the children. The children were able to differentiate voiced and voiceless sounds such as "s" and "z" and "t" and "d" through the vibrating boxes. Those with the most severe hearing loss responded to the vibrator boxes with speech sounds where no such speech sound had existed, and two children developed better voice quality (eliminating the high-pitched voices). All fifteen children were able to initiate stressed and unstressed syllables which is necessary for the teaching of proper speech melody.

INTENSITY INDICATOR: The intensity indicator is a visual aid to indicate the intensity of speech and covers a range from 20 decibels to 100 decibels. This is from very soft, to normal, to very loud speech. All fifteen children learned to control the intensity of their voices to some degree. This is accomplished by the child speaking into a microphone which produces a light at various intensity, with the teacher indicating the desired degree of loudness. With minimal instruction (first exposure), the children were able to grasp this concept and correct intensity.

SELECTOR: The selector is an amplifier for use with children with less severe hearing loss who do not require highly selective filter amplification. It is possible with the selector to provide group instruction (up to eight children) with different types of hearing loss from moderate to severe. The children using the selector are able to switch from one channel to another, depending on the speech sounds being emphasized. The selector has a maximum of 40 decibels amplification whereas the filter is able to amplify up to 120 decibels. The children who used the selector were able to discriminate between voiced and voiceless sounds and were able to hear word beginnings and word endings not heard through their own hearing aids. It was observed by the teacher that children were more careful in their pronunciation so as to include the word beginnings and word endings. This has not been observed in their speech prior to instruction on the selector.

Eighteen children were enrolled in the summer program with 90 to 95 percent attendance during the four weeks that the equipment was available. Fifteen of these children are alluded to in the above sections. The three remaining children did not take part to any significant extent in instruction with the equipment. This included a two-year-old boy who was enrolled for diagnostic purposes, a fifteen-year-old new to our school system who has a hearing loss and who has always rejected her hearing aid and a seven-year-old, multi-handicapped child with severe psychopathology and who has no speech or language.

The fifteen children involved with the equipment responded with a high degree of enthusiasm throughout the entire period. With the younger children (five to eight years old) in particular, the attention span seemed to increase each day so that by the fourth week, attention was significantly improved over the first and second week. The above statements regarding changes in behavior as a result of use with this equipment becomes more significant in view of the fact that Miss Kain, the teacher, had worked with most of these children during the 1971–72 school year and had a thorough knowledge of the speech and language characteristics of each child. Baseline data is therefore obtained from the teacher's prior knowledge of each individual child.

There were definite gains in each child in this short period of time though longer exposure to instruction with this equipment is necessary in order to have the desired carryover into spontaneous speech. The equipment on display here has been purchased by the Superior Public School System, and we shall be able to continue with the program initiated last summer.

*   *   *   *   *   *

SUMMER ENRICHMENT FOR HEARING IMPAIRED CHILDREN––TITLE VI

Evaluation:

Introduction

This project was planned cooperatively by the Superior Public Schools, the Department of Public Instruction and Title VI, E.S.E.A. There were several objectives of this program, though the primary aim was to evaluate equipment designed by Professor Djordje Kostić and sponsored in the United States and Superior by the Psychology Department of the University of Wisconsin—Superior and the Indian Health Service, Washington, D.C. The program was initiated on June 19, 1972.*

Children

The Superior Public Schools operated three units in deaf education during the 1971–72 school year with a maximum enrollment of 24 students. When the program was developed, it was anticipated there would be

* Funding for this project was later extended to December 1972.

twenty students attending the summer classes, though actual enrollment in June was eighteen.

Fourteen of the eighteen had attended classes in Superior during the past year, with the remaining four including a two-year-old boy who was enrolled for early education for diagnostic purposes, a nine-year-old boy who has a long history of learning problems, including hearing impairment, who has never attended classes in deaf education, a seven-year-old girl who had previously attended classes in deaf education in Superior but was now integrated into regular elementary school and a fifteen-year-old girl with a significant hearing loss and serious learning problems who has always rejected amplification.

Five of the eighteen were nonresident children who attended classes in the public school program during the 1971–72 school year and who were able to attend the summer session when their parents made special boarding arrangements. Total summer enrollment included nine boys and nine girls with an age range from two to fifteen years. The range of hearing loss was from moderate to profound.

Staff

The six-week instructional program was under the direction of Miss Frances Kain, certified teacher of the deaf, assisted by Mr. Arthur Baker, provisional teacher of the deaf, and Mrs. Helen Schroth, teaching aide.

The Indian Health Service, in cooperation with the University of Wisconsin–Superior, sponsored by Professor Kostić, Director of the Institute for Experimental Phonetics and Speech Pathology, Belgrade and Dr. Spansenija Vladesavljevic, scientific fellow at the same institute in Belgrade, Yugoslavia. Rhea Das, Ph.D., Professor of Psychology at the University of Wisconsin–Superior, who was originally responsible for introduction of Professor Kostić and his methodology to Superior, coordinated efforts between the university and the Superior Public Schools.

Professor Kostić, originator of the methodology and instrumentation, was an active consultant during the four-week period. Dr. Spansenija Vladesavljevic instructed Miss Kain in the Kostić Methodology and in the use of the equipment.

The equipment, consisting of four units—filter, vibrator, selector and intensity indicator—was available to the University of Wisconsin–Superior on loan from the Speech and Hearing Center, University of New Mexico, Albuquerque and the Indian Health Service. This equipment, never previously used or demonstrated in the United States, had been purchased for use in the Speech and Hearing Center at the University of New Mexico. Because the University of Wisconsin–Superior was conducting a workshop separate from the Title VI project, the equipment was made available to the University of Wisconsin—Superior and placed at the Weisberg Memorial Center, Superior Public Schools, during the first four weeks of the summer program. Following this four-week period, the equipment was sent to New Mexico, where Dr. Spansenija Vladesavljevic instructed personnel there in the use of this equipment.

Procedures

The special equipment was installed in the Weisberg Memorial Center the week of June 12, 1972, prior to the first day of school for children on June 19. The original program design called for pretesting of all students the last week of the regular school term with an articulation test. Responses were taped; however, the quality was too poor to be used. Consequently, it was necessary to administer again the articulation test the first two days the children were in session, June 19 and 20. This was administered by Miss Kain, who had also previously administered audiometric tests to children who would be attending the summer session. Pyschometric evaluations, including the Leiter International Performance Scale, W.I.S.C., Bender Gestalt and Human Figure Drawing were obtained on fourteen of the children. Using results obtained from the speech articulation test, a speech program was developed and implemented for each child using the various pieces of equipment. For purposes of this project, each child received individual instruction with the equipment though small groups were also used periodically. This was continued each day until July 14th, the last day that the equipment was available. A post-tape articulation test using the filter was completed the last two days of the four-week session.

On July 17 and 18, a speech articulation post-test was taped under the same conditions as the pretest using the same word list. The remainder of the two week session was spent developing vocabulary for field trips to the zoo, airport, fire station and a picnic to Billings Park.

A qustionnaire was sent to parents asking their opinion of the program and their children's reactions.

Advisory Committee

An Advisory Committee, as outlined in the Title VI proposal, was established. This committee met five times during the duration of the summer school program and once following the six-week session. The committee consisted of two parents of hearing-impaired children attending the program, a rehabilitation counselor from the Division for Vocational Rehabilitation, a university professor from Superior and an education consultant from C.E.S.A. #1. Initial meeting with the committee was designed to acquaint each member with the purpose of the program and its objectives and to demonstrate the use of the equipment.

Media

One of the program objectives was to disseminate information to the general public. This was accomplished by periodic coverage from local T.V. stations, articles in the Superior Evening Telegram and presentations to local service groups.

Evaluation

The effectiveness of the equipment was evaluated by the professional staff immediately following the four-week period. Results were written up and forwarded to the Department of Public Instruction and Title VI Evaluation Consultant on July 17, 1972.

Advisory Committee Report

On July 13 the Advisory Committee met and discussed the results of this equipment. Miss Kain shared her observations and impressions. On July 20 the committee met again specifically to hear pre- and post-speech tapes and to discuss further results and implications. All committee members were favorably impressed with the reactions of children to the equipment. Two committee members who were parents reported that their children were enthusiastic about coming to school and that in each case their children, both boys, had displayed improved speech at home. For example, one parent noted that for the first time, her seven-year-old son was able to produce the "s" sound in calling his friend "Steven." After a lengthy discussion, the committee strongly recommended immediate purchase of the equipment so that it would be available to the children in September 1972.

Parent Evaluation

Upon completion of the six-week session, a questionnaire was sent out to each parent and boarding and foster parent. The results indicated unanimous support of the program, and in most instances, definite gains in speech by their child during the session.

Equipment Maintenance

One of the primary concerns with electronic equipment, especially that produced in other countries, is the durability and maintenance features. During the four weeks, a power-supply problem resulted in technical difficulties. Other than this the equipment did function without mechanical breakdown.

A consulting engineer was brought in to help the staff evaluate this equipment, and it was his opinion that the equipment was essentially well made and would not be difficult to maintain. Parts are available in the

United States. Also it would not be difficult to obtain an adequate power supply. In fact by the third week with the equipment, the power problem was solved.

Who Can Instruct With The Equipment

With approximately three weeks of training, a teacher of hearing-impaired children, with an extensive background in speech, should be able to effectively use this equipment.

Visitors

During the four-week session with the equipment, there were sixty visitors to the program, including audiologists, speech therapists, school administrators, Department of Public Instruction consultants, Board of Education members, parents and friends and representatives from the news media. In addition, the program was visited by forty students attending classes at either Wisconsin State University—Superior or University of Minnesota—Duluth.

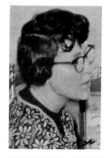

FRANCES KAIN

Miss Frances Kain received her undergraduate education in deaf education at Illinois State University, Normal, Illinois and has done graduate work at ISU and Wisconsin State University-Superior, Wisconsin. She taught hearing-impaired children on the primary, pre-primary and preschool levels in the public school system at LaCrosse, Wisconsin, from 1951–1969. She is in her second year with the Superior, Wisconsin, public schools, teaching hearing-impaired children on the primary level.

In the summer of 1972, Miss Kain worked with Professor Djordje Kostić, Dr. Rhea Das and Dr. Spasenija Vladesavljevic in a six-week instructional program for hearing-impaired children, using the instruments and methodology originated and developed by Professor Kostić.

Table XXI-I
TEACHER'S OBSERVATIONS

Name of Child	Selective Auditory Filter Amplifier	Vibrator	Intensity Indicator	Selector
1. Brenda Age: 7–8 Hearing Loss: Profound GROUP II	Worked with filter often to develop listening skills—learned to repeat *ma, bye, pa. ba* through listening.	Worked with v. boxes almost daily—learned to discriminate between *m, p* and *b* sounds and *f* and *v* sounds. Produced short and long *a*, short *i*, long *o*, *ai* and *ew*. Repeated *up, um, ma* and *pa*. Distinguished between loud and soft sounds. Could repeat correctly stressed syllables—*ma-Ma, pa-Pa*. Better voice quality.	Used seldom—needed work with filter and vibrator more. Was able to monitor intensity of voice when used.	Did not use—hearing loss too severe.
	Combined use of filter and vibrating boxes—*m* and *p* sounds—*papa, baba*			
2. Hans Age: 7–4 Hearing Loss: Moderate to severe GROUP III	Was able to produce initial *s* and *t* with vowels. Later got final *s* and *t* with vowels, *ch-, -tch, dr, st* and *z* and *th*, voiced and voiceless.	Could differentiate between *s* and *z* and *v* and *f*. Was able to reproduce *z* and *v* with vowels and *s* in word position, such as in word *voice*.	Used once—is able to monitor intensity.	Selector #4 —was able to produce *s, z, f, v, th¹, th², ch* and *-tch*.
3. Brian Age: 7–6 Hearing Loss: Profound GROUP II	Could produce *m, p, b, s* and *t* sounds. Got vowels: *ee* and *oo*. Could say *some, top* and *pie*. Got *s* in medial position. Voice was better with filter.	Could differentiate between *p, b, m-s, z*. Got vowels and diphthongs *a, e, ai, oo, oy*. Could repeat stressed syllables. Voice almost normal.	Used occasionally. Intensity better when using indicator.	Tried although hearing loss severe. #3—could repeat *t-, n-* and *d-* #8—could get *s* and *t*.
4. Jodi Age: 10–1 Hearing Loss: Moderate GROUP IV	Corrected or added *g-, ch-, -ch-, -ch, -tch¹-dz*. *-r* blends *dr, gr, thr, str* and word endings *-lm, -lt, -lk, -ng, -rd*. Used these sounds in words and simple sentences.	Differentiated between *m, b, p* and voiced and voiceless fricatives. Used short sentences to develop melody of speech.	Did not use—is able to monitor own intensity.	#3—worked on same sounds as with filter and got correct pronunciation.
5. Annette Age: 6–11 Hearing Loss: Profound GROUP I	Could produce *m* and *p* sounds with vowels *ah* and *uh*. Voice was a little better.	Worked daily with vibrator. could differentiate *m, b, p*. Could repeat *ah-m, up, um*. Voice was a little lower.	Used seldom. Needed work with filter and vibrator more. Could monitor intensity of voice when used.	Did not use—hearing loss too severe.
	Combination—Could repeat *m, p, b, um, up, ah, ahmah* and two and three syllables.			

Name of Child	Selective Auditory Filter Amplifier	Vibrator	Intensity Indicator	Selector
6. Bridget Age: 6–9 Hearing Loss: Moderate GROUP IV	Could produce s, z, f, v, k, g sounds with vowels in initial, medial and final positions. Could repeat two syllables. Got k and l sounds in names of siblings, *Colleen, Kelly* and *Kevin.*	Was able to differentiate between s and z, f and v and v and k and g.	Used seldom—is able to monitor own intensity.	#3 and #6 could articulate f, v, s, k and g sounds.
7. Arnold Age: 8–8 Hearing Loss: Severe GROUP II	Could produce m, p and b sound with vowels in all positions. Was able to repeat -f, -t, -t-, -d, d-, s- and -h. Finally got vowel ee with p sound in initial and final positions. Voice better. Combination—two syllable words— *mama, daddy, water.*	Could differentiate m, p and b and t and d. Better voice quality.	Seldom used. Needed work with filter and vibrator more. Could monitor intensity of voice when used.	Did not use. Hearing loss too severe.
8. Dick Age: 9–4 Hearing Loss: Slight to moderate. (other disabilities) GROUP IV	Was able to produce t-, sh-, -sh-, -sh, s-, v-, -l-, -th-, -ng, -d and r blends. ——	Seldom used. Has almost normal hearing in low frequencies.	Worked to decrease intensity of voice. Was able to increase and decrease intensity upon demand.	#3—could produce t, sh, s, and r blends. Could articulate correctly short sentences using these sounds.
9. Mike Age: 15–7 Hearing Loss: Moderate GROUP IV	Corrected or added d-, -t, -n, -i, r blends and word endings -nk, -lk, -lt, -ts, -ng. Was able to correct own speech through listening.	Used occasionally to produce better voiced sounds.	Used occasionally to increase intensity. Was able to monitor own intensity.	#2—could produce -n and d- words, word endings and words in sentences. #8—could produce fricatives and differentiate between s and z.
10. Billy Age: 7–7 Hearing Loss: Profound (Other disabilities)	Could produce ma, ahm, pa, up, bah, oo, ee and poo. Babbled into microphone. Combination—Could produce short duration vowel sounds.	Could differentiate between p, b, m. Could repeat ma, mama, ba and pa. Could differentiate between f, v; and prolonged ahhh and short ah; and soft and loud sounds. Babbled a great deal.	Used seldom. Needed work with filter and vibrator more. Could monitor intensity of voice when used.	Did not use. Hearing loss too severe.

(Continued on next page)

Table XXI-I (*Continued*)

Name of Child	Selective Auditory Filter Amplifier	Vibrator	Intensity Indicator	Selector
11. Denise Age: 10–10 Hearing Loss: Severe GROUP III	Corrected or added d-, s-, -s, n-, -n, -st, t-, r blends, k, g, ch, sh and dz sounds. Combination—Good differentiation in production of s and z.	Could differentiate between s and z. Could produce z with vowels.	Used seldom. Could monitor own intensity.	#8—could produce -s, -ch, -sh, -l- and dz and word endings.
12. Connie Age: 6–11 Hearing Loss: Moderate GROUP II	Could produce -g, -d, -ng, h- and wh- and s and z words. Got correct stress in two-syllable words.	Could differentiate between s and z and sh and zh sounds.	Used to increase intensity. Was able to produce normal and loud intensity.	#8—could articulate correctly r-, h-, -d, -g, -ng and s and z words. Could produce word endings in general conversation. Could produce sentence melody.
13. Eddy Age: 5–4 Hearing Loss: Severe GROUP II	Could repeat p, pee, papa, up, ma, mom, um, ahm, fah, ga-ga and ka-ka. Combination—Was able to say m, p, b sounds with ah, ee, ow and ŏŏ.	Could differentiate between p, b, m and repeat mama, papa and ahmah. Repeated loud and soft sounds and two and three syllables. Babbled a great deal.	Used occasionally. Was able to change intensity when asked.	Not used. Listening habits not well enough established yet.
14. Larry Age: 13–4 Hearing Loss: Moderate to Severe GROUP III	Corrected or added h-, -d, s-, t-, -t, st-, -st. Could produce these sounds with vowels and in words. Voice better. Combination—Better m-b and s-t discrimination.	Used to produce better voiced sounds. Could differentiate between s and z.	Used seldom. Could monitor own intensity.	#2—Could articulate correctly k-, g-, n-, -n, z- and r blends; and word endings -lt, -lk, -ch, -tch, -ng and -nk; and words and short sentences using these sounds. Voice better.
15. Cathy Age: 7–2 Hearing Loss—Severe to profound. (Attended only 7 times)	Could produce s in initial and medial positions. Responded to stimulus sounds below 455 Hz although audiogram indicates no hearing remnants below 500 Hz.	Used once—could discriminate between p, b, m.	Used once—could monitor own intensity.	#8—Could produce s sound.

YOUNG ADULTS
AND SUMMARY

YOUNG ADULTS

Dr. Griffiths: Throughout this Conference, when I received a great deal of attention and was given citations full of *whereas* phrases, those are, in my estimation, dividends as my friends in the stock market say. But the continuing satisfaction of working with children is my pleasure. To me, no Conference like this would be a success, if we did not hear from some of those youngsters. We had difficulty in narrowing it down. The HEAR Foundation youngsters, Mrs. Pollack's youngsters and San Diego Speech and Hearing youngsters—all of them—once they learn to talk, are very difficult to shut up. They are all eager to participate, and they have anticipated today with eagerness. We are very proud to present them to you.

I am having them in two sections, merely because we could not get them all on the stage, and we endeavored to divide them into age brackets.

Mrs. Muriel Taylor, who is a staff member of the San Diego Speech and Hearing Center, is going to take charge of the first section.

Their audiograms and their histories are arranged alphabetically, beginning on page 227. The first group is Wayne Olds, Joe Haggerty, Debbie Beck, Karen ReVeal and Linda McEwan.

Mrs. Taylor: Joe, would you like to introduce yourself?

Joe: Hello, my name is Joe Haggerty.

Mrs. Taylor: All right, would you give the microphone to Wayne, and we will have Wayne introduce himself.

Wayne: Hello, my name is Wayne Olds.

Mrs. Taylor: All right, let's give it to Debbie.

Debbie: My name is Debbie Beck.

Mrs. Taylor: Give it to Karen; would you introduce yourself?

Karen: My name is Karen ReVeal.

Mrs. Taylor: Linda?

Linda: My name is Linda McEwan, and I live in San Bernardino.

Mrs. Taylor: We are going to start with Karen and Debbie from San Diego, doing some discrimination, and then we are going to talk to the whole group. So, Karen and Debbie, do you want to come over here? Karen, do you want to hold the microphone for us? Debbie, you too. Come on. That's the spirit. You can both work at it at the same time. Now, because you are not going to be able to see what they are working at very well,

I'll read these sentences that we have. (The two children stood with their backs to the audience and Mrs. Taylor stood behind them.) "I ride a bike;" "I fly a kite." Why don't we go over it once so the audience will know what we are working with. "I talk in a mike;" "I ride a horse;" "I walk to a light." Okay, let's try it.

(Children pointed to appropriate sentences.)

Mrs. Taylor: I fly a kite. Right. I ride a horse. Right. I talk in a mike. Right. I walk to a light. No, I walk to a light. Right, Karen. Sometimes one of them get's it, and the other doesn't. I'll say: "right, Debbie" or "right, Karen." I talk in a mike. Right, Debbie. I ride a horse. Right, Debbie. I ride a bike. Right, Karen. I walk to a light. No, wrong. I walk to a light. Right, Karen.

Mrs. Taylor: Let's try the other one. Two girls go to a pool. Right, Debbie. The two girls go to the cool pool. Right, both of you. The girls go to school. Right, Debbie. The girl goes to the pool. Right, Karen. The girls go to the cool pool. Right. The two girls go to the cool school. Right. Two girls go to the pool. Right. The girls go to school. Right. Thank you.

Mrs. Taylor: Wayne, how did you get down here today?

Wayne: By airplane.

Mrs. Taylor: Did you fly PSA?

Wayne: Yes.

Mrs. Taylor: Was it on time?

Wayne: Yes.

Dr. Griffiths: Wayne, tell them where you live.

Wayne: In San Jose.

Mrs. Taylor: Would you tell us about the sculpture that you do?

Wayne: I don't do much.

Mrs. Taylor: O.K., you made something, didn't you?

Wayne: Yes.

Mrs. Taylor: What did you make?

Wayne: A submarine.

Mrs. Taylor: Tell me some more about it. Did you copy it from a book?

Wayne: No, I did not.

Mrs. Taylor: How did you make it?

Wayne: I designed it myself.

Mrs. Taylor: O. K. I wish I could do that. Let's give Joe a chance. Joe, what would you like to tell us about?

Joe: Well, I just don't know what to say.

Mrs. Taylor: Tell us about your interest in sports, how's that?

Joe: I am interested in sports. I am a sports enthusiast, whatever.

Mrs. Taylor: What do you like best?

Joe: Whatever is in season, everything.

Mrs. Taylor: What instrument do you play?

Joe: Pardon me?

Mrs. Taylor: Do you play a musical instrument?

Joe: Yes, the piano.

Mrs. Taylor: What kind of music do you like?

Joe: Well, I really haven't made up my mind about that.

Mrs. Taylor: Are you trying them all out?

Joe: Yes.

Mrs. Taylor: Do you try *rock* or *classical* or everything?

Joe: Well, I think so.

Mrs. Taylor: How about Wayne. What musical instrument do you play?

Wayne: The trumpet.

Mrs. Taylor: Do you have any particular kind of music that you like?

Wayne: Kind of fast.

Mrs. Taylor: Let's give the mike to Debbie. Debbie, what musical instrument do you play?

Debbie: What?

Mrs. *Taylor*: What musical instrument do you play?

Debbie: The organ.

Mrs. *Taylor*: What's your favorite song?

Debbie: "America."

Mrs. Taylor: You like "America" best. Where do you go to school?

Debbie: Parkway.

Mrs. Taylor: What's your favorite subject?

Debbie: Homemaking.

Mrs. Taylor: Karen, would you like the mike? Karen, how old is your new niece, Christine?

Karen: Five months old.

Mrs. Taylor: You like her, don't you. What's your favorite subject? Or your favorite class? What's your favorite class in school? What do you like best? This new semester you changed to homemaking?

Karen: Yes, homemaking.

Mrs. Taylor: Let's give the mike to Linda. Linda, do you belong to the Girl Scouts?

Linda: Yes.

Mrs. Taylor: How many badges have you earned?

Linda: Twenty-one.

Mrs. Taylor: That's great. Can you speak a little louder. You haven't often had this many people to talk to at one time. Can you tell us some of the subjects that you got your badges in?

Linda: Backyard fun, health services; I can't remember them all.

Mrs. Taylor: When you have that many badges, it is pretty hard to remember them all. I don't think we have that kind of auditory memory, most of us. What musical instrument do you play?

Linda: I play the organ.

Mrs. Taylor: Do you have a favorite song?

Linda: I forgot the name of it.

Mrs. Taylor: Well you probably have a lot of songs that you play, don't you? Where did you come from this morning?

Linda: I came from San Bernardino.

Mrs. Taylor: Great, was there much traffic?

Linda: No.

Mrs. Taylor: Being Saturday, you were able to get in on good time?

Linda: Right.

Dr. Griffiths: The next group of youngsters are in the young adult classification, and they too have come a long distance to be with us. The second group includes: Aleta Gruener, Gabrielle (Gigi) Gruener, Patty Jensen, Corinne Krahn, Don Liveley, Sherry Niemann, Tracy Plank and Linda Turner.

The chairman of this group is Mrs. O'Connor from Portland, Oregon. I really wanted to have somebody who was totally unfamiliar with the children and they with her in order to be able to show that communication is possible and relatively easy. Mrs. O'Connor.

Mrs. O'Connor: Thank you. I am in the same spot that you're in because I'm seeing some of the young people for the first time. When you come up here, you are just going to have to help me with your names. I met some of you earlier today. I think it would be interesting if we would tell the audience, or if each of you would tell the audience about your school experiences. How many of you are going to college now? Raise your hand high so that everyone can see. (Don Liveley, Tracy Plank, Corinne Krahn and Sherry Niemann raised their hands.) There are four of you. Then four of you are still in high school. How many of you are seniors? (Patty and Gigi.) Then we have one junior? I'm guessing . . . sophomore? (Aleta) Oh, sophomore. What do you do in school now, Aleta? Do you take part in school activities? Aleta, tell us something about your social life.

Aleta: I'm currently involved in gymnastics program, that is what I do, and I am on the team. I take five solid classes, I don't know what else.

Mrs. O'Connor: Do you get along well in the team?

Aleta: Yes, I'm getting high grades.

Mrs. O'Connor: Good. What do you do for social life; do you go out yet?

Aleta: I spend a lot of time with my friends. Most of the time I spend at the "Y" where I work out.

Mrs. O'Connor: How about you seniors? What are you doing now? How about you, Gigi?

Gigi: I am taking three special classes in school. I'm taking graphic art. I am taking food and nutrition and landscape occupation. My major field is in home economics. I intend to go to college and major in restaurant management for two years, and next I intend to go to Europe and go to a chef's school and become a chef.

Mrs. O'Connor: That sounds very exciting. Are you going to compete with Julia Childs?

Gigi: Yes, that is one of my main ambitions is to be like Julia Childs.

Mrs. O'Connor: O.K. How about you, Linda? Where do you go to school?

Linda: I'm in G. Jolly Geherten High School. I'm a senior, and my favorite class is art. I want to be happy because it's fun for me there. I like it here.

Mrs. O'Connor: Do you have very many dates?

Linda: Yes, I have many dates.

Mrs. O'Connor: Do you go out with hearing boys or hearing-impaired boys? Do you have other hearing-impaired students in your school?

Linda: I date both.

Mrs. O'Connor: Is there another senior? Patty, tell us about what has happened to you in the past couple of years. You said you moved. Tell us what your experiences were when you moved.

Patty: Well, we moved up to Vancouver, B.C. six and one-half years ago, and when I did move up there, I didn't think anyone had ever heard about hearing aids, so I was hiding them with my hair, and I wasn't telling my friends I wore hearing aids, and my teachers didn't know. Nobody knew until I said something or when my mom talked to some of the teachers about my school work, and they were flabbergasted . . . they didn't believe it. I had to show them the hearing aids and how they work, and they were interested in it. They accepted it. And it took me awhile to accept the fact that I wore them, and I am proud of them, and I thank Dr. Griffiths for all she has done for me.

Dr. Griffiths: I am very proud of you, Patty.

Mrs. O'Connor: That's good to hear, Patty. Don, how do you feel about your hearing aids? Did you have to come to some kind of a decision about your aids? Do you have anything to add to Patty's feelings?

Don: Well, she may think that there are people in the Canadian wilderness who don't know about hearing aids, but there are people in the great urban area in Los Angeles who don't because I still find them occasionally. I have never had to make any real decisions in so far as being limited. Anything I set my mind to, I felt that I could go ahead and do it without worrying about the fact that I have a hearing impairment. You know, I don't consider myself handicapped, in the sense that people think, "Well, he's deaf, he's handicapped." I don't. I can go out there and do everything that everybody else tries to do that doesn't have a handicap, etc. So I attempt to go out and reach the full potential and I don't say, "Well, I have a hearing loss, therefore, I can't." There's nothing like that at all. So that basically is what I can say at this moment.

Mrs. O'Connor: Patty, how about you?

Patty: No, it doesn't bother me. It used to bother me when I was younger. Little kids in elementary school don't know, and they are curious and they start making cracks about it and all this, but now it doesn't bother me anymore, because I have had the aids so long.

Mrs. O'Connor: How about you, Tracy?

Tracy: No, it didn't bother me. It makes me hear. It doesn't bother me and a lot of people, as Patty has said, were surprised that I was wearing hearing aids, and it doesn't bother me at all; it just helps me, and it is just a thing that I live with, and it's just very normal with me, and I had them since I was about four, and they are a part of me. I guess I just don't consider myself handicapped at all.

Mrs. O'Connor: Do you like to dance?

Tracy: Yes, I like to dance. I'm in college, and I do a lot of outside work activities. I am going to nursery school and working with small children, and I was in a sorority, and I've done some things in that. I am in an organization, a service organization for sophomore girls. It is a national organization, it is something like Red Cross Club. I would like to do service work for other people, and that's what I mainly do.

Sherry: Let me answer that question about hearing aids. To me, it is like putting on a pair of glasses, and I wouldn't be without them at all. I even wear them when I go to sleep because I am afraid I won't hear some things. You can't go without them. I get very upset when one of them isn't working.

Mrs. O'Connor: I think it's interesting that you wear them to sleep. Does it make a difference if you don't have them on? Does it wake you up if you don't have them on?

Sherry: Yes, I wouldn't hear the alarm unless I didn't wear one of them. I usually just wear one, though, when I sleep, and I trade off each night, you know. I sleep on this side, sleep on that side.

Dr. Griffiths: She wants to say something else because I see she has some notes.

Sherry: I only did this because I have a tendency to forget things. What I want to say, but I guess I will tell about myself, I hate to, but nobody knows who you are unless you tell about yourself. So . . . I am going to graduate school now, and we have audiology and I have a B.A. in Deaf Education. I entered the acoupedic program when I was four years old and have gone to regular schools and regular colleges since I was younger. This summer we started a group for hearing-impaired young adults, teenagers, who are coming up through the auditory program. The group is called ECHO, and we share experiences and problems because when a child, when a teenager gets to be older, he goes through an identity crisis, and he doesn't know whether he wants to be part of the deaf world or part of the hearing world. And he has to decide around the time he becomes a teenager . . . who am I, what do I want to do? On top of it, he has to decide whether he wants to continue in auditory approach or if he wants to go back and live in a deaf world. I think that by having this type of group, the only person who is going to be able to help them is someone who has been through this program, so mainly what we try to do is give him this kind of encouragement to go to an auditory approach. We started out with seven, and we now have twenty-five, but all of them did not go through the acoupedic program. They are oral, or whatever you want to call it; most of them did not come from the acoupedic program, but I feel that even though they are teenagers, they still have the same problems. Being oral, whatever.

Don: I would like to relate an experience I saw yesterday between two young ladies. They are in this group that is up here today. When they first met each other, they both looked at each other, and they both thought that neither one was wearing hearing aids, and when they both spoke, they felt the same way, and I had to introduce each one and say, "She is going to be in the program." One girl said, "You're going to be in the program—do you wear hearing aids?" This is the point that we're trying to achieve here, that there is a potential for normalization, whereas these two youngsters that I mentioned were considered profoundly deaf and there was no hope given for them when they were about age three and four, etc. So you can see that for some there is great potential. And when you look at some of the things that are going on elsewhere, I just have sat back in utter amazement that people still put their head in the sand.

Mrs. O'Connor: Well, we're going to get their heads out of the sand, Don. How about you, Tracy, have you got anything that you would like to talk about? What are you doing in school and what activities?

Tracy: Well, I am trying to get into the X-ray technician program at Cabrillo. It is going to be really hard because like 50 students start out, and they only take about eight students every two years, so I am hoping. I have a lot of outside activities, and I belong to a lot of clubs. I go out a lot; I'm a gymnastic freak.

Mrs. O'Connor: How did you get in the club? Did you just join like all the rest of your high school students?

Tracy: No. You have to get accepted. You have to be like them; you have to believe like they do. It's mostly like volunteer community action.

Mrs. O'Connor: I was thinking of how you got involved in school activities.

Did you have trouble, did you have to learn to kind of make yourself known to the rest of the student body?

Tracy: O.K. I go to high school right now, and most of the kids by the time they reach high school have matured quite a lot, and they accept us the way we are. And that's good, because it gives us more confidence, and I am sure if you looked at some of these kids sitting here, the way they were seven or eight years ago and look at them now and see how much improvement they have made, it is really encouraging. That's one thing I want to do when I get out of school; I want to work in speech and hearing and work with little kids and get them like this because it's good when you hear like this and hear what everybody says and like they would like to go into speech and hearing themselves, and it's good because the best teachers are the ones who experienced the thing that they are teaching themselves. Like in school right now, more than half the kids I know don't know I wear hearing aids. They don't because I spend most of my time lip reading, and when they do find out, they ask me dumb questions like is that why I wear pigtails all the time, and I say no. But they treat you like a normal kid, they know that you don't want to be treated with sympathy: "I'll treat you as best as I can." You want to fit normal with society, you don't want to be above or below. And that's good, and a lot of my friends respect me for that and I respect them.

Sherry: It is good that some of us are going into speech and hearing and deaf education. When I went through college to get a degree in deaf education, I had to learn sign language to get my certificate and after all these years being through an auditory approach, the only way I could get my certificate was to learn sign language. I think it is good, and I wish more of us could get into this field, but some professionals in the field don't think we can do anything. So we have to cross their paths first, before you can even get in.

Mrs. O'Connor: I thought maybe we might take time to see if there were any questions from the audience. We've got about 15 minutes, I think,

————: Yes, I would like to ask a question. So often when you kids do well, professionals say, "Well, of course you're very exceptional; you must be very bright." Do you take that as a compliment? How do you feel about people talking to you like that?

Aleta: I don't feel special at all; sometimes, in a way, I feel put down because they think if you have a hearing problem, you are below everyone else, and that's not true. Because right now I am taking five, solid advanced classes, and I'm getting B's and A's in them. I work hard to get it, but when people say, "Oh, you must be a brain," it is not true. Just because we have a hearing loss, it doesn't necessarily mean that we are not capable of getting good grades like everyone else.

Gigi: I often heard people say, again and again, "but now it is time to change." We're not back in the 1950's or the 1960's when people thought someone with a handicap of some kind, a missing arm or leg, was considered "Wow, that guy must be really weird, or something of the sort." But now times have changed so much, they accept this as a general fact; they say, "Oh well, she wears a hearing aid, so what!" It's just like wearing glasses, like she said. It is just so normal. I may have to ask a person to repeat something once or twice because I don't understand them. Because there are some people I have to get used to, certain voices are clearer than others. After several years when you get the hang of lip reading, you can do it right off the bat, and you can understand them; sometimes it's had. It makes you feel kind of good to do something well.

Don: There was one comment I want to make. Aleta made a comment earlier, that kind of went along with what you were saying. Kids accept you as being normal because you act normal, and that's a testimonial in itself.

Dr. Griffiths: Any more questions?

Molly Holly: I'm Molly Holly, President of C.A.P. I have a question to direct to Sherry. Too often our successful oral children are lost into the mainstream. Sherry, how did you find the teenagers for ECHO? Was this formed while you were still in secondary school, or if you were in your regular school, how did you find the kids, and how did you keep them together? We talk about ODASS members, there are so few, but I think it is because these people are lost. They lead normal lives; they don't need an organization. How did you build it?

Sherry: We found these kids that were integrated in a regular school. We just started with seven of them, and seven of them knew other kids. They just keep multiplying. It is not hard to keep them together, if you have things to share in common. Like we go bowling or we play miniature golf or we have a picnic and a Christmas party. And we involve not only them, but their families, their other brothers and sisters, the whole family. We get together sometimes as a group, but mainly it is involvement with the outside world. I don't know if that answered your question.

Doreen Pollack: I would just like to make a comment about this because I know this ECHO group, and I think one of the great things that has been very impressive to the adults who have been observing this group is the fact that ECHO really was for expressing concern and help to others. I have kind of forgotten your motto now, Sherry, but anyway, they truly do this. Just from the outside looking at them, they have two concerns: One is for the younger children in our program, and they do tremendous things to help our younger children really get together once in awhile because in an individualized program, our young children don't have the kind of group experiences that some of you are used to, when you think about hearing-impaired children in groups in school. But they also, I was very pleased with the president of the group, he said, for the next two months we are going to have fun among ourselves. And that's great.

Dr. Griffiths: Any other questions? Somebody earlier said to me, could it be possible that in this Conference, we could pull together the fact that you just don't teach children to articulate, that they also have to think. Can anybody here question that these youngsters don't think? Having a meaning for communication is a way of expressing thought, and I think each youngster here has expressed thought.

I want to thank each and every one of you, Aleta, Gigi, Patty, Corinne, Don, Sherry, Tracy, Linda and Mrs. O'Connor.

Don: I wanted to make one comment, so far as I am concerned. Now, I think everybody up here is wearing two hearing aids, and I want to explain that I am not wearing two hearing aids because I can't at the moment, but if I could, I would be. So I have a particular problem with my left ear, so it prevents me from wearing an amplified sound in that ear. So I don't want any of you out there to think that I am sponsoring a monaural type of hearing system. O.K.? Thank you.

Dr. Griffiths: Don was fitted with two hearing aids and wore two hearing aids until about three months ago when this problem developed in his ear.

Sherry: O.K. I just want to say something to anyone here who is interested in the field but not really in it. I suggest you try it because I have had a taste of helping children before. In the sixth grade I helped a second grader be able to speak easier and to be able to talk to everybody, and I also improved their speech in about three months. And I tell you that it is one of the most satisfying experiences to actually help a child be able to communicate with others. I tell you if any of you here would be interested in doing something like that, I really suggest you do it as it is really a great experience, when you really help someone.

Gigi: I just have one special thing to say. Hearing is almost like a special gift; if you are deaf, you have learned something more than someone else. If you lip read, you can do something that they don't even know. You can keep them guessing. But it is really a special gift. It may sound weird, but it isn't all that bad, you get so used to it that you feel that you have something more than other people have. Like the blind, they have a sense of touch that you will never have for quite a long time. They know, and so do we. Thank you.

Mrs. Muriel Taylor: I wondered if Corinne would tell us some of the things she has done in San Diego with the school district and at college.

Corinne: I am not sure what you were referring to.

Mrs. Taylor: I am referring to your school visitation and your efforts to convert a number of people.

Corinne: It is on the other side . . . on the manual side. I had an interview with the man who is in charge of all the handicapped programs in the elementary schools in the District of San Diego. He was very interested. He had heard about me, and I had an interview with him, and he gave me permission to observe some of the classes for the deaf. One class I observed, they taught sign language and in another they tried it integrated, more orally. They were kind of hesitant about me, they didn't know quite what to do with me because I went through the program at the HEAR Foundation. But I observed and I want to see if I could work on a project on HEAR Foundation, independent project for college, as a class to try to prove that it is a more valid approach, that it is possible for a deaf child with residual hearing to be able to hear and to be able to talk normally with hearing aids. The visitation of these two classes in San Diego has really made me want to work all the harder to prove that they need to be taught orally, the way I have been taught. I feel very sad about it because they didn't have very good training; I am not trying to criticize them, but I am just trying to say objectively that they need to be trained a little better. It has just really opened my eyes and I just want to prove that it is not the HEAR Foundation kind of help. I would put it that way.

Tracy: I just wanted to say that we need people like you and Dr. Griffiths. I give my special thanks to her because without her, there is no me. May I just say one more thing? Well, we talk too much, but I just want to tell you people that I am really glad that you all came to this Conference because it made me feel better to know that all of you care about and believe in an auditory approach. I hope that something will come out of this Conference and you will get together, forget your professional rivalries or whatever, and just work together. Because I know how hard it is to come up against someone that tells you "you can't do it" or "why are you doing it," so I just hope that you will work and put it all together. All of us, I think you will agree with me, we're only limited now in the goals that we have set for ourselves.

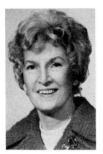

KATHRYN O'CONNOR, B.A., M. Ed., M.A.

Kathryn O'Connor did her undergraduate work at University of Washington, Seattle, received her Masters in Education, majoring in special education with emphasis on Education of the Deaf from Seattle University and a M.A. from Columbia University, in addition to which she has done continuing graduate work in teaching children with neurological impairment and other communication disorders at Washington University, St. Louis, Missouri. She has taught in regular classrooms for eight years before going into the area of education of the hearing-impaired. Her work with teaching hearing-impaired children ranges from nursery classes through high school. She taught for one year at Central Institute for the Deaf and was educational consultant for A.G.B. for two years.

Mrs. O'Connor was consultant for the School District of Washington, D.C., classes of multiple handicapped children, one of which was composed entirely of deaf-blind youngsters.

At present, Mrs. O'Connor is supervisor of a Department for the Hearing-Impaired in Highline School District which is a suburb of Seattle. Among her papers are: "Social Aspects of Integration," given at the International Congress on Education of the Deaf, Stockholm, Sweden, 1970 and "Maximum Integration for Severely Hearing-Impaired Students at the First Grade Level," given at the Alexander Graham Bell National Convention, Chicago, Illinois, 1972. She is a charter member of the American Organization of Educators of the Hearing-Impaired, Council for Exceptional Children, American Speech and Hearing Association, Washington Speech and Hearing Association. She is also a member of the Governor's Committee on Employment of the handicapped.

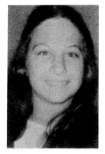

PURE TONE THRESHOLD AUDIOGRAM

This audiogram is plotted on the basis of:
☐ 1964 ISO reference thresholds
☐ 1951 ASA reference thresholds

NAME ___BECK, DEBBIE___

By ___San Diego Speech and Hearing Center___

CODE	LEFT EAR BLUE	RIGHT EAR RED
AIR	X	O
BONE COND. W. MASKING	◄	►
D B EFFECTIVE MASKING		
S. R. T.	70	70
M. C. L.		
T. D.		
P. T. A.		
S D S		

DEBBIE BECK (13) attended elementary school with hearing children. She is now in the 8th grade at Parkway Junior High where she is integrated into several classes each day and spends the rest of the day with the hard of hearing class. She is her class representative for student government; works as a student assistant in the office; and is a teaching aide in her P.E. class. She assists her mother at the Merle Norman Cosmetic Studios. Her duties are to help with the paper work and clean up after the complexion care. She has now become proficient enough to help the customers. She has a busy and varied social life; is active in her church; cooks and sews; and baby sits her twin sisters who are 2 years old. They are hearing children but Debbie has given them good auditory training. Debbie has taught herself to play the organ and has real musical talent.

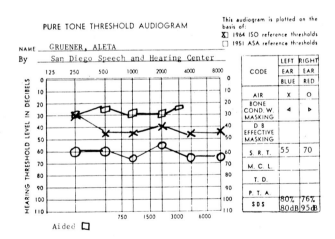

PURE TONE THRESHOLD AUDIOGRAM

This audiogram is plotted on the basis of:
☒ 1964 ISO reference thresholds
☐ 1951 ASA reference thresholds

NAME ___GRUENER, ALETA___

By ___San Diego Speech and Hearing Center___

CODE	LEFT EAR BLUE	RIGHT EAR RED
AIR	X	O
BONE COND. W. MASKING	◄	►
D B EFFECTIVE MASKING		
S. R. T.	55	70
M. C. L.		
T. D.		
P. T. A.		
S D S	80% 80dB	76% 95dB

Aided ☐

ALETA GRUENER (16) was 7 when she was fitted with aids at HEAR Foundation and has also pursued her education in regular schools. She is now a junior at Mission Bay High School and plans to attend college following her graduation to become a teacher.

227

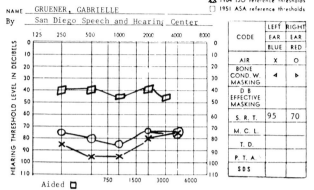

PURE TONE THRESHOLD AUDIOGRAM

This audiogram is plotted on the basis of:
XX 1964 ISO reference thresholds
☐ 1951 ASA reference thresholds

NAME GRUENER, GABRIELLE

By San Diego Speech and Hearing Center

CODE	LEFT EAR BLUE	RIGHT EAR RED
AIR	X	O
BONE COND. W. MASKING	◄	►
D B EFFECTIVE MASKING		
S. R. T.	95	70
M. C. L.		
T. D.		
P. T. A.		
S D S		

Aided ☐

GIGI GRUENER (17) is the eldest of three sisters all of whom were fitted with aids at the same time at HEAR Foundation in San Diego. Gigi was 8 at the time. She has gone to regular schools and is now ready to graduate in June from Mission Bay High School. She plans to attend the California State University at Santa Barbara to study to be a restaurateur and to do follow-up studies in Europe.

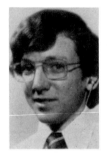

PURE TONE THRESHOLD AUDIOGRAM

This audiogram is plotted on the basis of:
☒ 1964 ISO reference thresholds
☐ 1951 ASA reference thresholds

NAME HAGGERTY, JOSEPH

By HEAR Foundation

CODE	LEFT EAR BLUE	RIGHT EAR RED
AIR	X	O
BONE COND. W. MASKING	◄	►
D B EFFECTIVE MASKING		
S. R. T.	85	95
M. C. L.		
T. D.		
P. T. A.		
S D S	90%	65dB

Bi Aided ☐

JOE HAGGERTY, 14 years old, entered the HEAR Foundation at the age of 3 years and 3 months. Etiology: Rubella. He was equipped with binaural aids and came for lessons twice a week. He attended regular nursery school until he entered Mark Keppel in Glendale in an integrated program. From the 3rd grade on he was in regular classes all the time. He was a Little Leaguer. He completed 7th and 8th grade at Wilson Junior High (Glendale). He is in the 9th grade at Loyola High which was achieved by competitive examination. His hobbies are chess, intramural sports, and reading. He plays the piano, has a daily paper route and is particularly interested in mathematics. Joe's hearing aids have been especially modified for wide range amplification by an uncle.

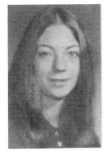

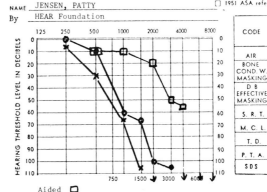

PURE TONE THRESHOLD AUDIOGRAM

This audiogram is plotted on the basis of:
☒ 1964 ISO reference thresholds
☐ 1951 ASA reference thresholds

NAME JENSEN, PATTY

By HEAR Foundation

CODE	LEFT EAR	RIGHT EAR
	BLUE	RED
AIR	X	O
BONE COND. W. MASKING	◄	►
D B EFFECTIVE MASKING		
S. R. T.		
M. C. L.		
T. D.		
P. T. A.		
S D S		

Aided ☐

PATTY JENSEN (17) was in kindergarten before her hearing loss was ascertained. The ski-slop loss enabled her to hear voices; the unintelligible speech was thought to be an attention getting factor as she had a very ill brother. She entered the HEAR Foundation at 5½ years of age and gained all her education in the regular public schools. The family moved to Vancouver, B.C. where Patty graduated from elementary school and is now a senior in the Lord Byng Secondary School and will graduate in June. She started piano lessons when she was seven years old and the piano teacher said she was the most promising student she had in her twenty years of teaching piano. Her hobbies are sewing and reading and the activities of Job's Daughters. When Patty was eight she could sing perfectly all the tune and all the words of "Supercalifragilisticexpialidosius" and thought Dr. G was pretty tongue tied not to be able to do likewise!

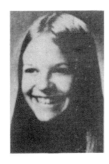

PURE TONE THRESHOLD AUDIOGRAM

This audiogram is plotted on the basis of:
☒ 1964 ISO reference thresholds
☐ 1951 ASA reference thresholds

NAME KRAHN, CORINNE

By San Diego Speech and Hearing Center

CODE	LEFT EAR	RIGHT EAR
	BLUE	RED
AIR	X	O
BONE COND. W. MASKING	◄	►
D B EFFECTIVE MASKING		
S. R. T.	70	75
M. C. L.		
T. D.		
P. T. A.		
S D S	80% 90dB	92% 90dB

Aided ☐

CORINNE KRAHN (19) entered the HEAR Foundation program at the age of 4½ years. Her family moved to San Diego from Canada to gain help for Corinne but she was not fitted with aids until she started at HEAR. She attended private nursery schools and private elementary schools through the first four years. Corinne also has had multiple health problems and had one kidney removed when she was about six. One of the ways that her mother helped her through the post-surgical hours was to have her aids put on and talked to her so that she wouldn't be as frightened. When Corinne was in high school, she won a contest for selling the most subscriptions among 150 competitors. She also was in need of major surgery again and yet she graduated from Patrick Henry High School with honors enough to win four scholarships to college. She was awarded a four year scholarship at Linfield College in Oregon where she is now in her second year.

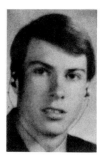

PURE TONE THRESHOLD AUDIOGRAM

This audiogram is plotted on the basis of:
☒ 1964 ISO reference thresholds
☐ 1951 ASA reference thresholds

NAME LIVELEY, DONALD
By Otologic Medical Group, Inc.

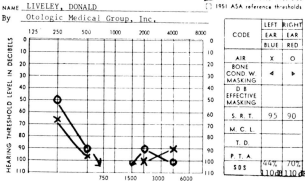

CODE	LEFT EAR	RIGHT EAR
	BLUE	RED
AIR	X	O
BONE COND. W. MASKING	◄	►
D B EFFECTIVE MASKING		
S. R. T.	95	90
M. C. L.		
T. D.		
P. T. A.		
S D S	44% 110dB	70% 110 dB

DON LIVELEY, 22, was diagnosed as totally deaf and mentally retarded when he was three years old. At four he entered the HEAR Foundation program and said his first word on the day he was fitted with aids. He attended regular nursery school and from then on gained his education in the Los Angeles regular public schools. He graduated from Wilton Place Elementary School and went on to Hamilton High from which he graduated in 1969. He was on the track team in Hamilton High, maintained a 3.0 grade average and participated in an advanced placement European history program for which he received college credit. He entered the De Molay at th age of 17. In 1968, he was the De Molay Master Councillor of the Lawrence C. Kelley Chapter and received the Past Master service award the same year for his outstanding performance. In 1971, he received the Southern California De Molay of the Year award and the same year was presented with the Distinguished Service Award for all around development. He has received the Chevalier Award, the highest honor received by a De Molay member and served as Vice President of the Western De Molay Region. He is now the Associate Advisor with the Council of De Molay Lawrence C. Kelley Chapter. He attended Pepperdine University for a year and is now a senior at the University of Southern California.

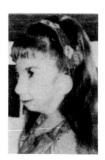

PURE TONE THRESHOLD AUDIOGRAM

This audiogram is plotted on the basis of:
☒ 1964 ISO reference thresholds
☐ 1951 ASA reference thresholds

NAME McEWAN, LINDA
By HEAR Foundation

CODE	LEFT EAR	RIGHT EAR
	BLUE	RED
AIR	X	O
BONE COND. W. MASKING	◄	►
D B EFFECTIVE MASKING		
S. R. T.		
M. C. L.		
T. D.		
P. T. A.		
S D S		

LINDA Mc EWAN (12) was born five weeks prematurely with a variety of anamolies. At first thought to be deaf and blind, she began to respond visually after 5 or 6 days and to respond to some auditory signals, too. And then the mother was told she was normally hearing. By the time she was 4½ years old, she had a few words in her vocabulary and was judged mentally retarded. She entered the HEAR Foundation program in San Bernardino at that time, was fitted binaurally, and due to the obstructive component, made rapid progress. At the end of the first year, she had learned to read and was in a regular school program in which she has continued and is now in the 6th grade at Parkside Elementary School. Over these years, Linda has been in surgery innumerable times, for her eyes, for her heart, for her ears. About a year ago, during surgery, it was necessary to perform a tracheostomy which will remain until all plastic surgery has been completed. Meanwhile, Linda has been active in Girl Scouts, likes to sew, and to play the organ.

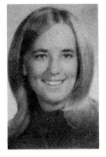

PURE TONE THRESHOLD AUDIOGRAM

This audiogram is plotted on the basis of:
☒ 1964 ISO reference thresholds
☐ 1951 ASA reference thresholds

NAME NIEMANN, SHERRY

By Porter Memorial Hospital, Denver Colorado

CODE	LEFT EAR	RIGHT EAR
	BLUE	RED
AIR	X	O
BONE COND. W. MASKING	◄	►
D B EFFECTIVE MASKING		
S. R. T.		22
M. C. L.		
T. D.		
P. T. A.		
S D S		

72% 40dB
Bi Aided

SHERRY L. NIEMANN was born Sept. 15, 1949 in Denver Colo. Her hearing loss was not discovered until age three when her speech was not progressing. After psychological testing which was inconclusive, she was taken to an ear doctor who had to be convinced of a hearing loss. After removal of infected tonsils and adenoids at age four which alleviated some of her conductive loss, she was found to have a severe bilateral sensori-neural hearing loss. The ear doctor then told her parents she would never be able to talk. Further diagnosis showed she also had athetosis as a result of an Rh negative blood factor existing in her mother at the time of birth. Sherry was fitted with a hearing aid at age four and attended for a short time the Denver University Speech and Hearing Clinic and then went to Evans School until age eight. She then entered a regular school, University Park Elementary School, at third grade. At age 12, she entered Thomas Jefferson Junior/Senior High School and graduated in the top one third of her class. During these high school years she was involved in many activities. She was a member of the Pep Club; Atherfies, a girl's honor service organization, active in Girl Scouts, was a Junior Escort, won two awards her senior year, Crisco Award — Outstanding Senior Girl in Home Economics and for Junior Achievement — Secretary of the Year.

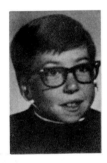

PURE TONE THRESHOLD AUDIOGRAM

This audiogram is plotted on the basis of:
☐ 1964 ISO reference thresholds
☐ 1951 ASA reference thresholds
1969 ANSI

NAME OLDS, WAYNE

By Ear Medical Clinic of Santa Clara Valley

CODE	LEFT EAR	RIGHT EAR
	BLUE	RED
AIR	X	O
BONE COND. W. MASKING	◄	►
D B EFFECTIVE MASKING		
S. R. T.	60	50
M. C. L.		
T. D.		
P. T. A.		
S D S	88%	84%
	85dB	85dB

WAYNE OLDS (12) entered the HEAR Foundation program at 2 years of age. He was born with a hearing loss, partial cleft palate and achondroplasia. The family at that time lived in Santa Barbara and traveled to Los Angeles twice a week for lessons. When he was old enough for school, he was able to go to regular school. He has had major surgery on his back and during that convalescent period had a home tutor. When she was explaining the physiology of hearing to him and was saying: "You hear with your ears," he corrected her. "No," he said, "I hear with my hearing aids." Wayne is now in the 7th grade of Piedmont Middle School in San Jose. His hobbies are sculpturing, reading and playing the trumpet.

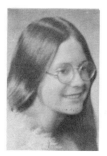

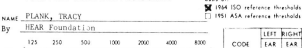

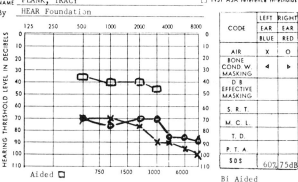

TRACY PLANK (17) was born with normal hearing but was stricken with meningitis when she was three years old. Her hearing loss as a result was severe and the first assessment at two other centers was that the loss was total and that amplification was of no importance. By the time Tracy was four, her voice was affected and the final consonants were disappearing from her speech. She was enrolled in a pre-school class for the deaf in Glendale. She entered the HEAR Foundation program one year from the time she lost her hearing. She was fitted with binaural aids which she wore constantly from that time on. The next week when she was brought for her lesson, she refused to enter the building for fear her aids would be taken away from her. After her own aids were purchased she came happily for lessons. From the first grade on, she was in regular school, graduating from the D. J. Dedgwick Elementary School in San Jose. She graduated from Watsonville High School in June 1972 with a 3.5 grade average. She belonged to the Pep Club and tried out as cheer leader. She also tutored an emotionally disturbed girl and won an outstanding merit award for her work. She plays the piano very well. Her hobbies are writing and skiing. She is now in her first year at Cabrillo College and is trying to decide between teaching and X-Ray technician as a vocation.

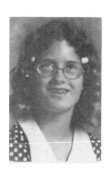

LYNN REINHARDT (12) entered the HEAR Foundation program at 2 years of age. She accepted her two aids from the time she was fitted. By the time she was ready for kindergarten, her language was extensive but her speech still not too clear. However, the regular school in Lakewood accepted her and she was tutored by a speech therapist to augment her school work as well as continuing at the HEAR Foundation until she was six years old. She continued in regular school and in the 5th grade at 10 years of age was moved into the accelerated program for Mentally Gifted Minors. She is now in the 7th grade in Roosevelt Junior High School in Lakewood. She reads and reads (anywhere from 8 books a week up) and is particularly interested in art. She loves to swim and plays baseball and basketball. On the family camping trips she collects rocks and does some rock polishing.

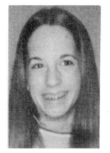

PURE TONE THRESHOLD AUDIOGRAM

This audiogram is plotted on the basis of:
☒ 1964 ISO reference thresholds
☐ 1951 ASA reference thresholds

NAME RE VEAL, KAREN

By San Diego Speech and Hearing Center

CODE	LEFT EAR BLUE	RIGHT EAR RED
AIR	X	O
BONE COND. W. MASKING	◄	►
D B EFFECTIVE MASKING		
S. R. T.	100	95
M. C. L.		
T. D.		
P. T. A		
S D S		

Aided ▢   Aided SDT 40

KAREN ReVEAL (13) attended regular elementary school and is now at Chula Vista Junior High. She maintains a regular class schedule with hearing children and goes to the hard of hearing teacher who functions as a resource teacher and counselor. During 5th and 6th grades, Karen was a library assistant and a student aide in the kindergarten. She attended San Diego Ballet School classes where she was commended for her good performance. Last summer she was solely responsible for the housekeeping at home which involved a certain amount of concern for her younger brother. Karen is an excellent cook and good manager. She is an active member of Job's Daughters, Bethel 164, and has learned the ritual. She participates in her church activities, has been a Brownie, attends school sports events and has been a team captain in her P.E. class. She enjoys helping with her new niece, Christine.

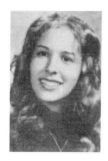

PURE TONE THRESHOLD AUDIOGRAM

This audiogram is plotted on the basis of:
☒ 1964 ISO reference thresholds
☐ 1951 ASA reference thresholds

NAME TURNER, LINDA

By HEAR Foundation

CODE	LEFT EAR BLUE	RIGHT EAR RED
AIR	X	O
BONE COND. W. MASKING	◄	►
D B EFFECTIVE MASKING		
S. R. T.		
M. C. L.		
T. D.		
P. T. A		
S D S		

Aided ▢

LINDA JEAN TURNER (17) entered the HEAR Foundation program at two years of age, came for lessons for five years, and has repeatedly returned to HEAR Foundation for progress evaluations. She attended private school (Faith Baptist School in Canoga Park, California) but entered the public school system when the family moved to Seattle in 1971. She is now a senior at King's Garden School, Seattle, and will graduate June, 1973. A recent evaluation at the Seattle Hearing and Speech Center reports: "Hearing levels revealed a severe to profound hearing loss. On the vowel discrimination task, Linda was able to achieve 58% correct at either ear monaurally and a 75% binaurally. With the 'Utley Lipreading Test', Linda was unable to understand any of the test questions through the visual sense alone; however, utilizing the test with my mouth and face obscured, Linda was able to understand quite well. This again supports the impression that most of her understanding ability is coming through the auditory channel." Linda's hobbies include a high interest in art (macrame, clay painting) and sports. Upon her graduation, she plans to attend business school.

CONCLUDING REMARKS

Dr. Stewart: During the time that this group was talking, one of my colleagues leaned over to me and said something, and I think I agree with him wholeheartedly. He said, "I wish I could talk that good." I don't mind their being able to speak so well, but I am disturbed that they don't show any nervousness because I do, even after having talked a number of years.

The people I have talked to around in the hall, while this has been going on, even before the last presentation, have said the same sort of things to me that I have been saying to myself: that I have been to a number of conferences over a number of years, and I have yet, until this time, gone away with the feeling of such nearly total satisfaction, delight, intellectual stimulation, than I have leaving this one today. If I can be forgiven a very bad pun, I did not come here to praise Ciwa, nor to bury her except maybe with one more accolade and again, Ole Bentzen is a very tough act to follow. I think what he said so well last night said what every one of us felt, that to elaborate on that would only do disservice to his statement. So I will just say that I go along with that wholeheartedly.

When the first brochure came out regarding this Conference, my first reaction was, "I think Ciwa has bitten off a larger chunk than any of us can chew in the time available to us." Once again it is a pleasure to get up and say how wrong you can be. She started off saying that we were going to cover at least four areas or four dimensions of an auditory approach, which I will give you very quickly: (1) early intervention with early amplification, (2) full time use of that amplification, (3) concern for the environmental factors, including appropriate equipment and (4) special techniques in methodologies to develop auditory processing. I think that this Conference has been much more comprehensive than this. For example, we have had some excellent exposure to some very basic research, particularly in areas outside our own, which I think has been very helpful.

The work on vision which was reported to us and the implications for people involved in hearing loss was tremendous. The work on the presentation on the genetic aspects of hearing loss, I thought, was one of the most clearly defined and described presentation on genetics that I have ever seen. I thought perhaps for the first time I was getting an inkling of this business of genetics in its relationship to hearing loss. We have gone quite a gamut from basic research to some very profound philosophical considerations, balanced up with some very, very practical discussions and some excellent demonstrations. We have been exposed to new information, at least new to me, about the relationships among various neuralphysiological perimeters, including the links not only between the eye and the ear but the links between the brain, tongue and the ear.

But particularly significant to me was the opportunity to learn what is being done and what is being thought about in various places throughout the United States, as well as throughout the world. I think that all of these presentations had as an over-riding theme: that we are all sincerely committed to an auditory approach and feel that we need to do all we can to spread this approach even further than it is now. The terrific feeling that I had the first day that "MY GOD, I AM NOT ALONE ANYMORE!" was worth the trip here by itself.

This Conference has established for us that we do have the thinkers, we have the innovators, we have the research, we have the technology, we have the clinicians, we have the educators, and they are all on our side. I think that with this, we should commit ourselves to see to it that the response that this Conference has generated is repeated and amplified wherever we can repeat it and wherever we can amplify it, whatever way we can spread it, so that the benefits accrued during these two and one-half days may be shared by more people than are in this room. Particularly, I think that this is important if we can come up with an answer to the question posed at this time as a concluding remark. I think we have seen over the past two and one-half days just about where we are. I would like to ask now, "Where do we go from here?"

Does anybody want to visualize what they think we can do from this point on? It would be a shame if this Conference ended and this was the end of the accomplishments.

Mrs. Helen Beebe: I am Helen Beebe from Easton, Pennsylvania. I work in a private practice, and I do not have a professional hospital, clinic or school system to work with. There was a question that I commented on earlier in the Conference about what good does it do to come here and talk to each other and not have the voice of dissent as we had for example at Alexander Graham Bell where we had an open discussion between total communication people and ourselves. I think we would all agree that we do need to have audiologists and hearing aid companies collaborate and understand what we are doing for these children. I would say that you should go so far as to appoint a commission to visit not only the meetings, the chairmen and the presidents of the organizations in audiology and hearing aid companies and to show them that they do not have the slightest idea of the potential of their product and that they can do much, much more to help these children. Every child up there who did a beautiful job could do it easier with less strain if the hearing aid companies and electronics in general would put their heads together to give us something better to work with and something less expensive. The audiologists who also work hard and are dedicated should have more exposure to the children as they go through these programs as to what they produce. I will give just one example, which I think I mentioned the other night at the HEAR Foundation. Our difficulty is with children that do very well, who are sent back to the audiologist, saying could we have a hearing aid evaluation, David is doing very well, but perhaps he could do better; could you reevaluate the hearing aid fitting. Nine times out of ten we get the response, "He's doing very well as it is, leave it as it is," without trying other hearing aids or trying to help the child that is doing very well to hear in an easier way for him.

Dr. Ole Bentzen: It is a very difficult question to answer, "What way shall we go?" As I have tried to show in my luncheon speech the other day, I feel quite sure that it must be a very broad approach. We have talked, and that is very nice and that is very important. We have talked about deaf children, but we have to talk about the deaf and hard-of-hearing population and in helping the whole population, we will include the children. I too have shown that one of the greatest resistants, to my mind or to my superior's, is such a simple thing—that we do not have mass production of hearing aids. The world production of hearing aids today is not over two million pieces, and we have 70 to 100 million people in the world who cannot hear. We have to focus very clearly. In an article that I have just finished together with my colleague, we have said in the last sentence that what we need is a uni (universal) aid, and, we think, a united nations' hearing aid. I think we have a great need to come to such a level. I could add that, being a medical person very happy to be here, in Denmark you cannot qualify as an otologist unless you have three months of work in an audiological clinic. We tried this some years ago through the Association of the Deaf in America to have that formed like the United Nations, but the doctors were pushed down because we were too few. Though I am not much for resolutions, ask Dr. Griffiths to find a man, and I know she knows him, who would be able to go into that business, telling people in the United Nations and elsewhere in the welfare, social work and political departments in Washington, D.C., that this is another way to go. Thank you.

Doreen Pollack: I would like to make one suggestion, that in every meeting that we have in the future, we let the young people take the lead because they are the people living with this problem. For too many centuries we, the normal hearing, have been telling them what to do. We tell them that we cannot prove that in the audiological testing that two hearing aids are better than one. But they say no, we prefer two. I would like them to get up and take the lead in the future and that is why I have worked hard to get my former graduates going. We cannot stop working with them too, but the very moment they need us for social support, they do not need us for speech or lip reading or those things. In the teenage years, they need us to help them apply the more social skills, some of the subtle things that go on that they seem to miss. So we can help them, but they should be taking the lead, and that is what I would like to see in the future.

Dr. Stewart: Ciwa just made a comment while you were talking, Doreen, that this is really the first generation of these young people who have been able to speak for themselves, and they are doing an admirable job of it. Another comment in the back.

Mr. Thomas Kneil: I am Mr. Kneil from Wichita State University, Kansas. I would like to reemphasize the point that Dr. Sanford Gerber made earlier, that we need documentation and evidence of the gains that are being made in the various areas that one's studies are in or investigation is in. That is, I have heard comments that in the clinic, we have not been able to demonstrate the benefits of the binaural hearing aids and therefore, there are those who don't believe they are useful. On the other hand, here are persons who do say and can demonstrate outside of the clinic that binaural hearing aids are useful and superior to the monaural. Under these circumstances, it seems to be appropriate that you should be documenting this in whatever way you can, so that it is available in the literature for people to look at and criticize and talk about and, hopefully, eventually believe, if that appears to be the case and that is true not only in the area of binaural hearing, but in your various methodologies that you are talking about. If these children that are reached early do in fact have better language and better speech, let us document it. Thank you.

Dr. Victor Garwood: I would like to address myself briefly to your statement about getting together. It is no accident that we have not gotten together so far. The state of California, and I cannot speak for any other state, has embarked on some programs which I think just begin to show results. The first thing that happened, obviously in my state, was that the doctors got licensed and that eliminates any medical chicanery. In the state, we are somewhat backward about the other people involved. We have now certificated teachers of the deaf, perhaps some of their requirements are antiquated. I think you can probably observe from your participation here that a lot of the radical work is being done in institutions such as HEAR Foundation. This is the way it should be. This has got to filter down more positively to the schools, and one of the reasons that it has not been filtering down is that other people involved with your children and with you teachers of the deaf have had really no rights. Recently, in the last year, hearing aid dispensers in California became licensed. Now the minute they signed their name to the document, they theoretically got out of a soft shoe business, or suede shoe business I think they call it, where someone will come out to your home and fit you with a hearing aid when you don't need one.

There are clauses in the present law that protect children up to the age 16; why it stops at 16, I could never quite figure out, but at any event they call for a combined evaluation from an otolaryngologist, which may in some respect be a step towards what Dr. Bentzen required in Denmark, and an audiologist. There are movements afoot right now to eliminate that from the law because it is inconvenient to certain hearing aid dispensers. The third thing that has happened in the state of California, and I would hope that it would be happening in other states, is that although it took us $20,000 to do it, speech pathologists and audiologists have been licensed. This doesn't answer the problem entirely. I think that if you have been paying any attention here today, all of us who are audiologists, and I am one, will realize how little we got in our training about the deaf and severely hard-of-hearing, but a new breed is growing. I do not know if Dr. Jeffers is in the audience today, but she has been battling for years trying to get educational audiologists, school audiologists, or whatever you want to call them—people who are attuned to the needs of children of school age and pre-school age, to be licensed. That will be coming, but you see that cannot come really, until audiologists are licensed in the first place. Now I think that when we start fulfilling what you are talking about in cooperation for the first time in the state of California, we will have a lot of problems because we will all be taking our vested interests with us. But believe me that when you stand up and have to take an oath that you are not an audiologist, not a hearing aid dispenser, not a physician, but you are acting in the public interest, a lot of your ideas begin to change. So I think, Dr. Stewart, we are just about to the threshold, but not quite. Thank you.

Mr. Bill Uebersetzig: I am Bill Uebersetzig. I work for the HEAR Foundation, but I would like to make my comments as a parent of a deaf child rather than as an employee of HEAR Foundation.

I, also, received a feeling of a great affirmative movement from this Conference. It has been positive all the way, and I am very excited about it. I think that one thing that my wife, Jan, and I have talked about and that we are committed to as a result of the Conference is that *Parent Power* is very important and that we realize that unity throughout the United States at least, and internationally also, can come about from this Conference. It would greatly spur on the efforts and the goals that we are working toward. I can understand the need for scientific documentation and the desire for clinical proof and various data that the educational field might require, but I think we might be able to speed that up a little bit with some unified *Parent Power.* I am going to commit myself, and I know Jan feels the same way to correspond with other parents. I was greatly encouraged by the listen program that we heard about at the HEAR Foundation on Thursday evening that is going on in Colorado. I think that is fantastic, the work that they are doing. I think that the rest of us parents throughout the United States, by corresponding with each other and pulling together, can really make it work and maybe speed the whole thing up a little bit.

Mrs. Mary Ann Burns: I am Mary Ann Burns from Helen Beebe's clinic in Easton, Pennsylvania. I wanted to comment on a point made the other day that I do not feel was satisfactorily answered, and I would be very disappointed if we left such a distinguished meeting as this without having at least acquired some kind of a directory of services regarding where the auditory programs are for parents to write to. Now I believe that at this point, Dr. Northcott mentioned that through the Alexander Graham Bell Association, they do have such a listing but the title given to the listing was oral programs rather than auditory programs. I feel that at too many of the meetings some of the representatives of the oral adult deaf section are not representative of auditory program products. For many new parents that go to these meetings, they do not see such a beautiful collection of individuals, as we were all fortunate to see today, of the young people that spoke today. Many of the parents, I feel, are scared away by some of the products they see there. I think that we must have a separate directory of the auditory programs because as even one of the deaf teenagers mentioned today, there is all the difference in the world in an auditory program and an oral program.

Mrs. Betty Petersen: In answer to your question, Joe, I would like to say that educationally, I think that Dr. Griffiths, Mrs. Grammatico, Dr. Ling, Doreen Pollack and Lois Tarkanian have shown us the way to go and I think that we can all help the electronic people. They have already made great strides in the last few years to be shown the way to go, but we need to have the medical people now to look at some other areas, biomedical perhaps, neurophysiological and then I think all of us, teachers, educators, medical people and audiologists, need to look at the whole child, not just an ear. Thank you.

Dr. Priscilla Muir: I am Priscilla Muir and I have already had a chance to talk to you, but I want to say once again what I said the other day. I think more than anything else what we need in this business is optimism and that I feel has been the real outcome of this Conference. We tend very often to look at the children who are not presently doing well through their ears and throw up our hands in horror. We have to find a way to get to those, and we can do it. I think we must have the optimism and the belief that this is the way to go. I want to make one other comment, we have not talked a great deal in this Conference about the relationship between audition and cognition. I happen to believe that must be the thrust of the future, for audition without a lot of meaning is not worth very much at all.

Dr. Stewart: I do not see any more hands up, so I will turn the meeting over to Dr. Griffiths.

Dr. Griffiths: I would just like to say goodbye, drive safely, fly safely; come back again to visit us. We will be in communication with each and every one of you because we want to keep this going. Thank you very much for coming.